Contents

Heart Failure Palliative Care

A team approach

SECOND EDITION

Edited by

MIRIAM JOHNSON

Professor of Palliative Medicine
Deputy Academic Programme Training Director
Hull York Medical School

CRC Press
Taylor & Francis Group
6000 Broken Sound Parkway NW, Suite 300
Boca Raton, FL 33487-2742

International Standard Book Number-13: 978-1-910227-35-0

Visit the Taylor & Francis Web site at
http://www.taylorandfrancis.com

and the CRC Press Web site at
http://www.crcpress.com

Printed and bound in Great Britain by
TJ International Ltd, Padstow, Cornwall

Foreword

Worldwide, heart failure is highly prevalent and, although the treatment of patients with heart failure has significantly improved during the last decades, prognosis remains poor. Heart failure is considered equivalent to many malignant diseases in terms of symptom burden, mortality and suffering. Heart failure is a progressive disease with an often unpredictable course, accompanied by many contacts with a broad array of healthcare providers. Since the release of the first edition of *Heart Failure and Palliative Care: a team approach* in 2006, there has been increasing discussion about the role of palliative care for people with heart failure. Professional heart failure guidelines and consensus papers advise provision of palliative and supportive care concurrent with efforts to prolong life. Increasingly, cardiology and palliative care professionals seem to be working together to optimise care.

During the patient's journey, people with heart failure and their families are often faced with several problems that require a broad, multidisciplinary approach and input from physicians, nurses and other healthcare providers; hence the need for a team approach.

A 'team' can be defined as 'a group of people who work together' and 'teamwork' as 'work done by several associates with each doing a part but all subordinating personal prominence to the efficiency of the whole'. But what is needed for optimal teamwork?

One of the issues to consider is the optimal composition of a team or, in other words, finding the best building blocks. There has been some academic discussion on who should be considered core members of a team, who should have a consulting role, who should have the lead and who should be responsible for coordination in palliative care? Should the cardiologist be/ stay in charge, should the heart failure clinic keep the coordination or should the primary care be central? If we put the person with heart failure and his/ her specific needs at the centre, these discussions become irrelevant. A 'team' does not have to be static or the same for each patient. There is no 'one size fits all' team composition. Depending on patient needs, historical and current roles of professionals, cultural issues and available resources, team members can be invited or consulted. Several collaboration models can be relevant in heart failure care – for example, in-hospital or home-care heart failure teams, palliative care services or hybrid models. Team composition may also change when the severity of heart failure progresses over time and patient needs and caregiving demands on family and caregivers intensify. The inclusion of family members or other care providers in such a team is a relevant crucial issue, and raises the question of whether professionals can see patients and their families as equal team members.

Another important aspect in optimal teamwork is mutual goal setting and open and clear communication. Mutual goal setting, designing a treatment plan and regular discussion of changes in goals of treatment and care are a vital feature in teamwork. Team members who care for heart failure patients often face the challenge of managing multiple conditions requiring multiple medications and lifestyle changes in persons who are sometimes cognitively and psychologically affected. An open discussion about goals that are relevant for the patient is needed to optimally diagnose, carefully review and prescribe treatment, and provide support to patients and families. Across the course of their heart failure, most patients will go through several phases that can be marked by different goals for treatment and care and different issues in communication. Patient and carer preferences may change as health status and other circumstances alter and should regularly be reviewed. Even with an unpredictable trajectory, it is vital to regularly evaluate the goals of treatment and care, as previous goals can become unrealistic and reflect false hope.

This second edition of *Heart Failure and Palliative Care* is an asset for all teams involved in the care of patients with heart failure, and it can be seen as the basis for optimal care. To deliver optimal care during the changing patient journey, healthcare professionals need to stay informed about new developments, be aware of evidence-based strategies and be informed about new approaches. The first edition of this book was received very positively by healthcare providers as one of the first heart failure-specific books about palliative care that addressed useful theoretical and practical knowledge. Its pragmatic approach opened the eyes of many 'cardiology people' and clarified the importance and relevance of palliative care for their heart failure patients. It also opened the eyes of many 'palliative care people' to the complexity of heart failure and the need for an interdisciplinary team approach. This second edition of *Heart Failure and Palliative Care* has the same pragmatic and realistic approach and has been updated with the latest evidence and insights. In this edition, palliative care for heart failure patients is placed in a wider international context and patient experiences and advance care planning are further elaborated.

In the Foreword to the first edition, Robert Twycross, Emeritus Clinical Reader in Palliative Medicine, Oxford University, wrote: 'Although much still needs to be done, there is definitely light at the end of the tunnel'. Since then (2006), a lot has happened with regard to palliative care for heart failure patients. Although we are not there yet, there are many international initiatives to improve care for patients with heart failure using a palliative care approach.

Tiny Jaarsma
Professor in Nursing Science
Linköping University, Sweden
Editor-in-Chief, *European Journal of Cardiovascular Nursing*
July 2015

Preface to the second edition

Famous last words: 'We really ought to update the book – it won't take long . . .'

Despite continued sales of the first edition and an ongoing and humbling number of people who have contacted us one way or another to say that, as we had hoped, this book had stimulated joint working between heart failure and palliative care professionals in their localities, we became painfully aware that it was not only very UK-centric, lacked anything about heart failure with normal ejection fraction and didn't say much about cardiac devices, but was also now very out of date. This latter point was one of rejoicing; palliative care for people with heart failure was clearly on the healthcare agenda and the field had progressed.

In this second edition, we have tried to preserve the ethos of the first – that is, that the book should be a clinical guide to help clinicians caring for people with advanced heart failure develop a team approach for a group of people who, despite the increased awareness, remains disadvantaged in accessing support to help them live with, and support them as they die from, this serious illness.

Again, when possible, we have tried to be evidence based, and we have been pleasantly surprised that there has been more published literature to discuss and include than we thought (hence 'famous last words'): no chapter could be left alone. Conversely, although we are pleased to have added a section in the first chapter about the evidence for palliative care for people with heart failure and that there are now several ongoing Phase III randomised controlled trials to evaluate effectiveness, we are disappointed that none of these are ready to be reported as level 1 evidence in this edition.

However, there were notable other encouragements. The first was that, since the first edition, Dr Karen Hogg had been appointed as the UK's first cardiologist with a special interest in palliative care – indicative of the growing recognition of the importance of palliative care in cardiology – and was therefore invited onto the editorial team. The second was that it was apparent that there were both strategic and clinical team changes to support an integrated approach to palliative care for people with heart failure around the world. Therefore, not only was it clear that we should invite a range of authors from around the world to contribute but also the last chapter on services needed to be almost completely rewritten. ('It won't take long . . .').

Like the first, this edition has been written by doctors and nurses who are clinicians first and academics second, if at all. The editors hold to their premise in the first book:

> Looking after end-stage heart failure is not rocket science. It is much more difficult. The trajectory of a rocket is predictable; the course of heart failure is not. Patients are not made of metal, and it matters what happens to them.

However, the changes that are apparent since 2006 show teams working together, getting on with the job to address the concerns and needs of these flesh and blood patients, and of those who love and care for them amidst the uncertainty and lack of clear prognoses.

However, there is still a way to go until palliative care for heart failure is an assumed part of routine care. We still need leadership and innovation on a wide scale. We need a continued change of attitude in primary care and secondary care through education and modelling of good practice by senior clinicians. Our continued hope is that those reading this book will be inspired to look at local ways to address the inequity of access to supportive and palliative care for patients with heart failure.

At the end of the Preface of the first edition we wrote, 'We hope that a future book might describe a very different picture as the research base of symptom control and service provision develops over coming years.' We are pleased that this hope has been realised enough to have made this second edition a much longer labour of love than we had anticipated. We look forward to a future edition that will tell a story of level 1 evidence and the systematic integration of training and practice to deliver services so patients do not have to have cancer before they can access excellent palliative care.

Miriam Johnson, Richard Lehman and Karen Hogg
July 2015

About the editors

Miriam Johnson, MD, FRCP, MRCP, MBChB (Hons), is Professor of Palliative Medicine at Hull York Medical School, and is Co-Director of the Supportive care, Early diagnosis and Advanced disease (SEDA) Research Group at the University of Hull and the Yorkshire and Humber Clinical Academic Training Programme Deputy Director. Her clinical and research interests include the palliation of breathlessness and palliative care for patients with advanced heart disease. The projects employ a wide range of research methodologies (clinical trials of drug or complex interventions, qualitative, observational, secondary data analysis, data linkage) and collaborative partners are involved across different disciplines and countries. She has published widely in her field and holds grants from a variety of bodies (National Institute for Health Research [NIHR], National Health and Medical Research Council [NHMRC], Dunhill Medical Trust, Marie Curie Cancer Care / Cancer Research UK [CRUK], Yorkshire Cancer Research, British Heart Foundation).

She is a member of the National Cancer Research Institute (NCRI) supportive and palliative care clinical study group and palliative care specialty joint lead for the Yorkshire and Humber Comprehensive Research Network. She holds clinical sessions with St. Catherine's Hospice, and the York Foundation Hospitals NHS Trust in Scarborough, North Yorkshire and set up one of the UK's first integrated palliative care services for people with heart failure.

Richard Lehman, MA, BM, BCh, MRCGP, is a Senior Research Fellow at the Department of Primary Health Care at the University of Oxford. He was a full-time general practitioner in Banbury for 32 years. For the last 17 years, he has also written a weekly summary of the principal medical journals that is posted on the *BMJ* website. Since his retirement from UK general practice in 2010, he has worked on studies of the patient experience and has spent a year at Yale working with the Yale University Open Data Access (YODA) project, for which he remains a consultant to the group. He is currently also working with Dartmouth College on shared decision-making tools for use in primary care and on a number of related projects. He is Senior Advisory Fellow in General Practice at the UK Cochrane Centre.

Dr Karen J Hogg gained degrees in science and medicine from the University of Glasgow in 1994 and 1999, respectively. In 2002, she undertook a British Heart Foundation Junior Fellowship and went on to achieve a postgraduate doctor of medicine degree in 2007, also conferred by the University of Glasgow, for research into heart failure with preserved systolic function. Her subsequent specialist clinical training was based in Glasgow, and, in 2010, she took up the post of Consultant Cardiologist with a specialist interest in heart failure and palliative care, based at Glasgow Royal Infirmary. In this unique post, she is the clinical lead for heart failure in North East Glasgow and the cardiology clinical lead for the Caring Together programme (jointly funded by the British Heart Foundation, Marie Curie Cancer Care, and NHS Greater Glasgow and Clyde). She is also an invited member of the Heart Failure Association of the European Society of Cardiology Joint Task Force on Palliative Care in Cardiology.

List of contributors

CHAPTER 1

Merryn Gott
Professor of Health Sciences
Faculty of Medical and Health Sciences
University of Auckland
Auckland, New Zealand

Clare Gardiner
Senior Lecturer
Palliative and End of Life Care Research Group
School of Nursing
University of Auckland
Auckland, New Zealand

Emilie Green
Academic Foundation Year 2 Doctor
Barts Health NHS Trust
London, UK

CHAPTERS 2 AND 3

Shona Jenkins
Consultant Cardiologist
Glasgow Royal Infirmary and Stobhill Hospital
Glasgow, UK

CHAPTER 4

Amy Gadoud
NIHR Clinical Lecturer in Palliative Medicine
SEDA Research Group
Hull York Medical School
University of Hull
Hull, UK

CHAPTER 5

Wendy Gabrielle Anderson
Assistant Professor
Department of Medicine
Division of Hospital Medicine and
Palliative Care Program
University of California
San Francisco, CA, USA

Steve Pantilat
Professor of Clinical Medicine
Department of Medicine
Division of Hospital Medicine and
Palliative Care Program
University of California
San Francisco, CA, USA

CHAPTER 6

Scott Murray
St Columba's Hospice Chair of Primary
Palliative Care
Primary Palliative Care Research
Group
University of Edinburgh
Edinburgh, UK

Marilyn Kendall
Research Fellow
Primary Palliative Care Research
Group
University of Edinburgh
Edinburgh, UK

CHAPTER 7
Iain Lawrie
Consultant and Honorary Clinical Senior
Lecturer in Palliative Medicine
Director of Medical Education
(Undergraduate)
The Pennine Acute Hospitals NHS Trust /
University of Manchester
Manchester, UK

Suzanne Kite
Consultant in Palliative Medicine
The Leeds Teaching Hospitals NHS
Trust
Leeds, UK

CHAPTER 8
Hillary Lum
Assistant Professor of Medicine
Division of Geriatric Medicine
University of Colorado Anschutz Medical
Campus
Denver, CO, USA

David Bekelman
Associate Professor of Medicine and
Nursing
University of Colorado

Director of the Palliative Care Clinic for
Heart Failure
Eastern Colorado Veterans Affairs Medical
Center
Denver, CO, USA

CHAPTER 9
Hayley Pryse-Hawkins
Heart Failure Nurse Specialist
Harefield Hospital
Royal Brompton and Harefield NHS
Foundation Trust
London, UK

CHAPTER 10
Nathan Goldstein
Associate Professor & Director, Palliative
Care Program
Hertzberg Palliative Care Institute
Department of Geriatrics and Palliative
Medicine
Icahn School of Medicine at Mount Sinai
New York, NY, USA

Laura Gelfman
Faculty, Geriatrics Research Education &
Clinical Care Center
Geriatrics Research Education and Clinical
Care Center
James J Peters VA Medical Center
Bronx, NY, USA

Piotr Sobanski
Consultant in Palliative Medicine
Hildegard Palliative Centre
Basel, Switzerland

Patricia Davidson
Professor, Dean, School of Nursing
Department of Acute and Chronic Care
Johns Hopkins School of Nursing
Baltimore, MD, USA

Jane Phillips
Professor
Career Researcher
Centre for Cardiovascular and Chronic Care
Faculty of Health
University of Technology Sydney
Sydney, Australia

Philip Newton
Career Researcher
Centre for Cardiovascular and Chronic Care
Faculty of Health
University of Technology Sydney
Sydney, Australia

Acknowledgements

The editors would like to thank all our chapter authors for their contributions, which in every case involved the hard work of breaking new ground and making new connections. We would also like to acknowledge the contribution of Louise Gibbs, Michael Davies and Clare Littlewood, who wrote for the first edition but were not able to contribute this time; their work has formed the foundation for this edition.

Bringing the book together has involved time and effort that have inevitably been taken away from other activities, and we are grateful to our work colleagues for their kindness and understanding on occasions when this has been apparent. Finally, we would like to thank our families for their patience and support, without which this book could not have been completed.

List of abbreviations

6MWT	6-minute walk test
ACE	angiotensin-converting enzyme
ACP	advance care planning
ADL	activity of daily living
AF	atrial fibrillation
ARB	angiotensin receptor blocker
BNP	B-type natriuretic peptide
COPD	chronic obstructive pulmonary disease
CPR	cardiopulmonary resuscitation
CRT	cardiac resynchronisation therapy
CRT-D	cardiac resynchronisation therapy defibrillation
CRT-P	cardiac resynchronisation therapy pacing
DNACPR	do not attempt cardiopulmonary resuscitation
ECG	electrocardiogram
EF	ejection fraction
ESC	European Society of Cardiology
GSF	Gold Standards Framework
H-ISDN	hydralazine and isosorbide dinitrate
HFrEF	heart failure with reduced ejection fraction
HFSN	heart failure specialist nurse
ICD	implantable cardiovertor defibrillator
LBBB	left bundle-branch block
LVAD	left ventricular assist device
LVSF	left ventricular systolic ejection fraction
MI	myocardial infarction
MRA	mineralocorticoid receptor antagonist
NCRI	National Cancer Research Institute
NHMRC	National Health and Medical Research Council
NHS	National Health Service
NICE	National Institute for Health and Clinical Excellence
NIHR	National Institute for Health Research
NSAID	non-steroidal anti-inflammatory drug

NYHA	New York Heart Association
PC-ACP	patient-centred advanced care planning
RAAS	renin–angiotensin–aldosterone system
RCT	randomised controlled trial
SEDA	Supportive care, Early diagnosis and Advanced disease
SHFM	Seattle Heart Failure Model
SPC	specialist palliative care
UK	United Kingdom
USA	United States of America
YODA	Yale University Open Data Access

CHAPTER 1

The need for palliative care in heart failure

MERRYN GOTT, EMILIE GREEN, CLARE GARDINER, RICHARD LEHMAN AND MIRIAM JOHNSON

INTRODUCTION

Over the last 50 years, evidence has been repeatedly offered to show that people with heart failure experience comparable levels of palliative care need to those with cancer.[1] However, in most countries, they remain disadvantaged in terms of consistent access to specialist palliative care services and are often not adequately supported by health and social care providers. Specific concerns have also been raised that communication relating to prognosis and preferences for end-of-life care is limited, in turn limiting the opportunities that patients and their families have to determine the nature of the care they receive. The unpredictable nature of their illness trajectory is a particular challenge in meeting the end-of-life care needs of individuals with heart failure and has proved to be a major barrier to the optimum timing of palliative care provision.

This chapter provides an overview of the experience of advanced heart failure, highlighting key issues from the perspective of patients and their families. A comparison with advanced cancer underlines the substantial palliative care needs of patients with advanced heart failure; the impact of epidemiological and socio-demographic factors is also outlined. The chapter concludes by reviewing the current evidence base for palliative care for people with heart failure.

PART 1: THE EXPERIENCE OF ADVANCED HEART FAILURE

I just walk around here and I'm really shattered. You know, it's as much as I can do, I'm afraid that's the worst part of my illness that I cannot get out and do what I want . . .

Mrs P, aged 85 years[2]

Early studies of patient experience of heart failure were mainly conducted in the United States using retrospective data gathered from hospital records.[3,4] The first large-scale community study to explore palliative care needs in heart failure was conducted in the UK. Symptoms were measured through validated self-completion questionnaires administered every 3 months for 2 years, or until death.[5] Overall, the study concluded that quality of life for these patients was 'difficult and challenging'. Female sex, four or more co-morbidities, New York Heart Association (NYHA) class III–IV heart failure and depression (evidence noted in nearly half of the sample) were associated with a higher symptom burden.[2]

A subset of participants took part in semi-structured interviews to explore their experience of this high symptom burden and the effect it had upon their lives. These qualitative data confirmed that breathlessness and fatigue were the most common symptoms and that these had a substantial impact on activities of daily living. One participant described her morning routine as follows:

The worst part I think is getting up in the morning. It takes me ages . . . I think it's the tiredness that affects me most. I sit on the edge of the bed and I put my slippers on. Then I put one arm in my dressing gown and I've to rest before I can get the other arm in . . . then I've to sit on the bed a bit while I trot off to the bathroom . . . I just brush my teeth, wash my hands and then I've to sit on the toilet seat to get my breath back to pull the curtains back in the bedroom. And then after I've pulled the curtains back then I've got to sit down again on the bed . . . I just dread the mornings really.

Mrs T, aged 85 years[2]

This account points to the significant impact that heart failure symptoms can have on the lives of patients and is consistent with other reports that fatigue and breathlessness are the most frequently experienced heart failure symptoms.[6,7] It is therefore unsurprising that social isolation is one of the biggest problems reported by people with heart failure, with many saying they feel trapped at home by their symptoms.[8] This is likely to contribute to the high number of mental-health problems disclosed by people with heart failure;[9] an important consideration to address given that depression is associated with higher levels of mortality within this population.[10]

The stark impact of heart failure on quality of life can be seen from a general survey of the epidemiology of heart failure in the West Midlands,[11] where the overall effect of heart failure due to systolic dysfunction was measured using the Short Form (36) Health Survey. In all domains, patients with heart failure due to any cause scored markedly lower than the general population and, in most domains, lower than those with other chronic illnesses, mental or physical (*see* Figure 1.1).

Looking specifically at the last 6 months of life, we have evidence from studies in three different countries that the symptom burden steadily increases. A common feature of all these studies is that pain is a frequent and severe symptom in many heart failure patients who are near to death. In the Study to Understand Prognoses and Preferences for Outcomes and Risks of Treatments (SUPPORT) study, carried out in a number of US academic medical centres during the 1990s, 41% of patients were reportedly in pain in the 3 days before death.[12] A Swedish study carried out at the same time produced similar findings and commented that although numerous distressing symptoms were well documented by doctors and nurses, there was little evidence that they were being adequately addressed.[13]

Patients may have a limited understanding of their condition, with many attributing their symptoms to normal ageing rather than a life-limiting condition. This is likely to relate to reported poor communication about diagnosis and prognosis on the part of health professionals. In a qualitative study from the UK in 2002,[14] few patients reported having had a discussion with their healthcare providers about the likely course of their illness and none had been asked about their preferences for end-of-life care. The implications of this lack of forward care planning could be seen in accounts of high levels of interventionist care received in hospital settings up until the point of death.[15]

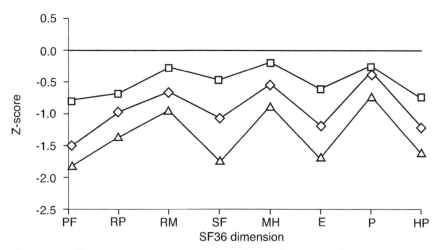

Z-scores of diagnosed heart failure patients divided into NYHA classes compared to the general population. PF = physical functioning; RP = role physical; RM = role mental; SF = social functioning; MH = mental health; E = energy; P = pain; HP = overall perception of health; — = general population; □ = NYHA class II; ◇ = NYHA class III; △ = NYHA class IV.

FIGURE 1.1 Quality of life in heart failure
Source: Hobbs et al.[11]

For example, the wife of a patient who died from heart failure in hospital describes his final hours as follows:

> She [the registrar] decided he needed a stomach x-ray because his stomach was very bloated but he couldn't eat or drink so she ordered this x-ray to be done. So less than an hour before he died, poor man, there were three of us trying to lift him onto an x-ray plate because obviously he had to go underneath. He was talking to me and I knew he knew he was dying.
>
> Wife, aged 47 years[15]

Similar findings regarding a lack of involvement of patients in decision-making have been reported in studies in other countries, with neither patient nor clinician being willing to address the 'elephant in the room',[16,17] highlighting the need for improved communication in heart failure as a priority (*see* Chapter 7, 'Communication in heart failure').

An understanding of what constitutes a 'good death' from the perspective of people with heart failure is crucial and should lead to tailored care for the individual within the context of their disease and stage of life. The philosophy of a good death, which underpins specialist palliative care (SPC) delivery, has been described as being pain-free and occurring at home surrounded by family and friends in line with personal preference and in a manner that resonates with a person's individuality, with death openly acknowledged.[18] However, there is evidence that this model of a good death, formulated as the foundation of the care of people dying with cancer, is not directly applicable to people with heart failure.[19] Heart failure predominantly affects older people and this has implications for the way the condition is experienced as well as the care and support required, particularly given the likelihood that patients will be experiencing co-morbidities and other physical and social challenges related to ageing. Further, many are aware of the risk of sudden death, and some within this group of patients may consider a sudden death, of which they are unaware, to be a good death, and preferable to a slower decline. As many already feel marginalised from society at this stage in life, they may be concerned that they are a burden.[19]

Trajectories and transitions

Patients with heart failure face an unpredictable disease trajectory, characterised by a gradual deterioration that is punctuated by acute exacerbations of circulatory inadequacy. The reasons for this erratic disease course include the widespread reversible pathological events superimposed on permanent structural changes, diversity in response to conventional therapy, progression of disease-modifying treatments and the impact of co-morbidities upon the individual.[20] Figure 1.2 provides an example of how the heart failure illness trajectory is typically represented diagrammatically.

The typical disease trajectory for cancer is thought to be different from that of heart failure. However, in studies of whole patient groups, these differences may be less extreme (*see* Figure 1.3).[22,23]

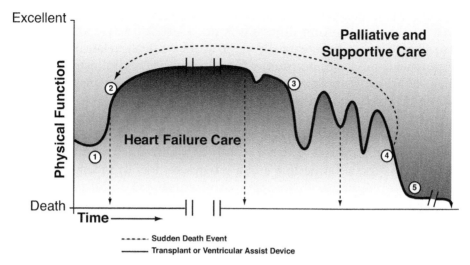

FIGURE 1.2 Heart failure trajectory[21]

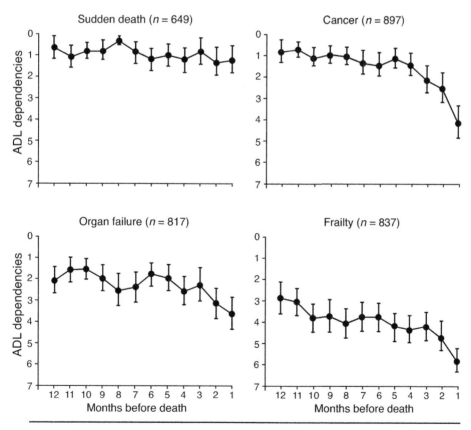

Error bars indicate 95% confidence intervals.

FIGURE 1.3 Group disease trajectories
Source: Lunney *et al.*[22]

Because quality of life is reduced and symptoms persist throughout the course of this life-limiting illness, it is necessary for active and palliative approaches to care to be integrated[21,24,25] to avoid a transition late in the disease trajectory with 'missed opportunities for palliation'.[26] This is illustrated by data from a UK primary care database study of heart failure decedents that showed that only 7% were entered on the palliative care register prior to death, and, of those that were, nearly one-third were entered within a week of death.[27] By comparison, half of cancer decedents were registered.

While the prognosis of patients with heart failure may be unpredictable, signs such as functional decline and a progressive loss of independence can indicate the need for a palliative approach.[28] Integrated and timely access to SPC should be available to patients with heart failure, but this does not happen consistently[29] (*see* Chapter 10, 'Palliative care services for patients with heart failure'). This is not only due to the unpredictable disease trajectory but also to patient and healthcare-professional characteristics, such as a focus on active treatment by cardiology specialists, the increasing age and number of co-morbidities of patients, poor communication with people with a non-cancer diagnosis and the lack of inter-professional education and clarification of roles among healthcare professionals.[30]

The UK's General Medical Council published guidance on end-of-life care defines 'patients at the end of life' as those likely to have less than 12 months to live.[31] Despite some predictive ability for the Gold Standards Framework (GSF) Prognostic Indicator Guidance for hospital inpatients of all diagnoses,[32] neither the GSF Prognostic Indicator Guidance nor the Seattle Heart Failure Index was helpful in identifying heart failure patients in the community with a prognosis of less than 12 months, although the GSF guidance identified those with significant symptom burden.[33] The challenges of predicting life expectancy may impair the appropriate involvement of SPC services or the adoption of a palliative approach to care by the usual team, despite the presence of a high symptom burden.[34] Therefore, a focus on patient needs/concerns, regardless of estimated prognosis, is preferred, which requires healthcare professionals to understand the patient's palliative care needs, build consensus within the clinical team as to how these should be addressed, successfully communicate the team consensus to patients and their families and regularly offer patients the opportunity to express and record preferences for end-of-life care that are subsequently acted upon.[35] The development and adaptation of a needs assessment tool designed to act as an aide-memoire in busy clinical practice has been validated for people with heart failure and may be a useful way forward if shown to make a difference to patient experience[36] (*see* Chapter 10).

Finally, a key priority must be to ensure that patients have adequate opportunity for autonomous decision-making throughout the heart failure trajectory, including with regarding to palliative and end-of-life care.[29,37] The involvement of patients and their families in decision-making, including eliciting their palliative care needs, is fundamental to providing this care.

Most people with advanced heart failure are older and many live with a spouse or partner on who they become highly dependent. There are limited data about the partnership status of heart failure patients, but the Manchester study found that 82% were married and living with a spouse, a much higher percentage than their cancer cohort.[38] The physical, mental and spiritual exhaustion that carers can suffer is well described in a review of the literature by Molloy and others.[39] The needs of heart failure patients who do not have a family carer are even greater. Some carers do not live with the person with heart failure and may not be so obvious to supportive services.

Heart failure and cancer compared

There are some striking similarities between the characteristics of heart failure patients and older cancer patients who already form the bulk of the palliative care caseload. McKinley and colleagues[40] looked at the records of 154 patients in two general practices in Leicester who died between 2000 and 2002. Of these, 108 died of cancer and 46 of cardiorespiratory disease. In both groups, the average age at death was 74 years, and there was no significant difference between the groups in terms of the number of co-morbidities.

Looking at the issues from a hospital perspective, the previously mentioned Manchester study was an important study was carried out in 1996 based in the first hospital clinic in the UK specifically for heart failure.[38] This compared the needs expressed by patients attending the heart failure clinic with those of patients receiving palliative care for cancer. Usefully, this study not only listed the symptoms experienced by the two groups of patients but also compared those that were perceived as most troublesome (*see* Table 1.1).

In the report of their study in Edinburgh, Murray *et al.*[45] provide a wide-ranging comparative analysis of main themes from interviews with sufferers from lung cancer and from heart failure (*see* Table 1.2).

These studies (*see* Tables 1.1 and 1.2) show that although the relative severity of symptoms can differ between heart failure and cancer, the total symptom load is certainly no lighter and may often be greater, with poorer access to supportive and palliative services.[46,47]

TABLE 1.1 Symptoms in cancer and heart failure in six studies[13,38,41–4]

Symptom	Cancer (%)	CHF (%)
Pain	35–96	41–78
Fatigue	32–90	69–82
Breathlessness	10–70	60–88
Insomnia	9–69	36–48
Anxiety/Depression	3–79	9–49

Note: Percentage ranges of patients in studies who experienced the given symptom.
CHF = chronic heart failure.

TABLE 1.2 Summary comparison of the experience of patients with lung cancer and heart failure

Lung cancer	Heart failure
• Cancer trajectory with clearer terminal phase. Able to plan for death	• Gradual decline punctuated by episodes of acute deterioration. Sudden, usually unexpected death with no distinct terminal phase
• Good understanding of diagnosis and prognosis	• Little understanding of diagnosis and prognosis
• 'How long have I got?'	• 'I know it won't get better, but I hope it won't get any worse'
• Swinging between hope and despair	• Daily grind of hopelessness
• Lung cancer takes over life and becomes overriding concern	• Much co-morbidity to cope with; heart often not seen as main issue
• Treatment calendar dominates life, more contact with services and professionals	• Shrinking social world dominates life, little contact with health and social services
• Feel worse on treatment: coping with side effects	• Feel better on treatment: work of balancing and monitoring in the community
• Relatives anxious	• Relatives isolated and exhausted
• Financial benefits accessible	• Less access to benefits with uncertain prognosis
• Specialist services often available in the community	• Specialist services rarely available in the community
• Care prioritised early as 'cancer', and later as 'terminally ill'	• Less priority as a 'chronic disease' and less priority later, as uncertain if yet 'terminally ill'

Source: Murray et al.[45]

Prognosis of heart failure and common cancers

Heart failure has often been referred to as a 'malignant' disease, with a prognosis worse than those of several disseminated cancers. This was strikingly demonstrated in a study by Stewart and colleagues,[48] who analysed data from all first hospital admissions in 1991 in Scotland for the commonest cancers and heart failure. The Scottish Morbidity Record Scheme was used to trace patients and calculate the 5-year survival for each cancer and for heart failure following first admission (*see* Figure 1.4).

In the Hillingdon study, similar results were obtained by comparing the survival of patients with incident heart failure with the survival rates for major cancers provided by the Office of National Statistics for England and Wales (*see* Figure 1.5).[49]

Although evidence-based therapies have had a positive impact on survival,[50] there is still a 3-year mortality rate of 25%,[51] and patients have a similar mortality, or worse, than for many types of cancer.[11] It is probably true that prognostic variability in heart failure is greater, but it is important to recognise that by the time a heart failure patient has required hospital admission, the risk of death in the next 18 months is over 40%.

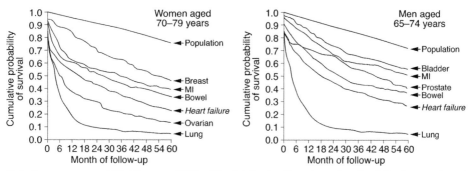

Data for women aged 70–79 years (28% of the total cohort) are based on the following number of patients: heart failure ($n = 1167$), myocardial infarction ($n = 1600$) and cancer of the lung ($n = 475$), breast ($n = 441$), bowel ($n = 369$) and ovary ($n = 108$). Similarly data for men aged 65–74 years (26% of the total cohort) are based on the following numbers of patients: heart failure ($n = 1063$), myocardial infarction ($n = 2083$) and cancer of the lung ($n = 1064$), bowel ($n = 485$), prostate ($n = 452$) and bladder ($n = 264$).

FIGURE 1.4 Age-specific probability of survival following a first admission for heart failure, myocardial infarction and the four most common types of cancer specific to men and women relative to the overall population
Source: Stewart *et al.*[48]

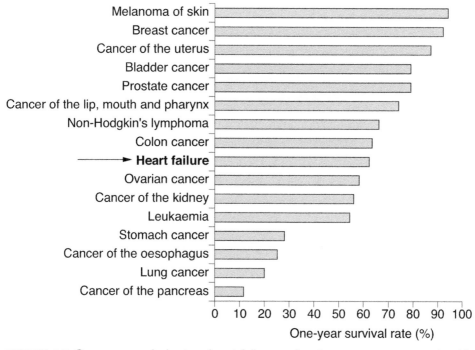

FIGURE 1.5 One-year survival rates, heart failure and major cancers compared, mid-1990s, England and Wales
Source: Cowie *et al.*[49]

Co-morbidity

It's just one thing after another, really. Which illness shall I start with?

Ms I, aged 78

The heart problem doesn't seem to be the thing that bothers us. The other illnesses are so obvious that her heart didn't enter the equation.

Carer of Mrs LL

Any patient with heart failure inevitably has co-morbidity (*see* Table 1.3), because 'heart failure' is not a diagnosis but the label used to describe the result of a disease process affecting the body's capacity to maintain an adequate

TABLE 1.3 Co-morbidities in a large US heart failure cohort study: 20 most common non-cardiac chronic disease conditions for patients aged 65 years or older with chronic heart failure (n = 122 630)

Chronic disease defined by CCS code	Per cent prevalence (n)
Essential hypertension	55 (67 211)
Diabetes mellitus	31 (38 175)
COPD and bronchiectasis	26 (32 275)
Ocular disorders (retinopathy, macular disease, cataract, glaucoma)	24 (29 548)
Hypercholesterolemia	21 (25 219)
Peripheral and visceral atherosclerosis	16 (20 027)
Osteoarthritis	16 (19 929)
Chronic respiratory failure/insufficiency/arrest or other lower respiratory disease excluding COPD/bronchiectasis	14 (17 610)
Thyroid disorders	14 (16 751)
Hypertension with complications and secondary hypertension	11 (13 732)
Alzheimer's disease/dementia	9 (10 839)
Depression/affective disorders	8 (9371)
Chronic renal failure	7 (8652)
Prostatic hyperplasia	7 (8077)
Intravertebral injury, spondylosis, or other chronic back disorders	7 (8469)
Asthma	5 (6717)
Osteoporosis	5 (6688)
Renal insufficiency (acute and unspecified renal failure)	4 (5259)
Anxiety, somatoform disorders, and personality disorders	3 (3978)
Cerebrovascular disease, late effects	3 (3750)

CCS = Clinical Classification System; COPD = chronic obstructive pulmonary disease.
Source: Braunstein *et al.*[53]

circulation. The commonest disease processes are ischaemic heart disease, diabetes and/or long-standing hypertension, and 90% of patients with heart failure have one or more of these. Benefit from heart failure treatment can be reduced by the presence of co-morbid disease – for example, diabetes.[52] The heart failure syndrome can, in turn, lead to other co-morbidities, such as depression, cognitive impairment or renal failure. Lastly, since heart failure is mostly a disease of old age, patients often have a number of unconnected health problems, such as cancer, osteoarthritis, hearing difficulty and/or macular degeneration.

The high prevalence of co-morbidity in heart failure (*see* Table 1.3), in common with the significant symptom burden, means that coordinated team effort is required to address the needs of most patients. The specialties with greatest expertise in this are primary care, palliative care and gerontology or general medicine, rather than cardiology. Notably, most cardiologists are aware of this.[54]

PART 2: PALLIATIVE CARE NEED
The size of the problem

When the need for palliative care in heart failure first became the subject of correspondence in the general medical journals,[55,56] a frequently expressed anxiety was that this would 'open the floodgates' and overwhelm SPC services. This has not been the experience of those palliative care services brave enough to have lowered their flood defences (*see* Chapter 10). As in so much else to do with heart failure, there are clearly complex factors at work.

BOX 1.1 New York Heart Association classification of heart failure

Class I
No limitations. Ordinary physical activity does not cause fatigue, breathlessness or palpitation.

Class II
Slight limitation of physical activity. Comfortable at rest. Ordinary physical activity results in fatigue, palpitation, breathlessness or angina pectoris.

Class III
Marked limitation of physical activity. Although patients are comfortable at rest, less than ordinary activity will lead to symptoms.

Class IV
Inability to carry out any physical activity without discomfort. Symptoms of congestive cardiac failure are present even at rest. With any physical activity increased discomfort is experienced.

Heart failure affects approximately 1%–2% of the population in developed countries. The prevalence is greatest among older people, rising to over 10% in those aged 70 years and older.[57] There are no UK epidemiological data on heart failure stratified by NHYA class (*see* Box 1.1), and the general quality of data relating to heart disease in the UK has been called into question by some epidemiologists.[58] Apart from the epidemiological uncertainties, it seems that social factors also play a major part in service use by heart failure patients.[59]

Ethnicity

Ethnicity is an issue that has received much international attention in the study of heart failure with regard to clinical factors,[60] even to the extent of recruiting specific ethnic groups to major interventional trials. However, data from the UK are scanty. Looking at ischaemic heart disease, which is the precursor of most systolic heart failure, there are wide variations between the main ethnic groups in England. The lowest rates are found in the Chinese and Black Caribbean populations, the highest in the Pakistani and Bangladeshi groups.

Heart failure has been found to present at an earlier age in South Asian men in studies carried out in Leicester,[61] Birmingham[62] and Harrow.[63] These studies do not conclusively show that the overall prevalence of heart failure is greater in South Asian immigrant populations, though this is likely. It seems that, in these groups, heart failure presents earlier and is associated with better survival.[64]

Mortality, mode and place of death

The system of death certification in the UK makes it hard to estimate the number of people who die from heart failure, because it may feature under the general label of 'ischaemic heart disease', or even as 'old age', as well as being recorded specifically as heart failure.

Death from heart failure can be sudden, due to electrical instability or a new ischaemic event, or slow, due to progressive organ failure and pulmonary oedema. All grades of heart failure carry an increased risk of sudden death, which usually happens outside hospital. Grade IV heart failure (NYHA classification) is the terminal phase, and, when such patients decompensate, their distress and breathlessness is such that they are almost always admitted to hospital. Therefore, studies of the mode and place of death in heart failure show a division between sudden deaths predominantly outside hospital and death from progressive heart failure ('pump failure') predominantly within hospital (*see* Table 1.4).

TABLE 1.4 Place and mode of death of heart failure patients in two major interventional studies

Study	In hospital	Out of hospital	Not reported
AIRE*			
Sudden	133	135	
Chronic HF	182	10	
Total	315	145	
ATLAS†			
Sudden	149	439	1
Chronic HF	309	97	39
Other	271	71	7
Total	729	607	47

Notes: *UK, post-infarction only; 45% of patients who died suddenly had severe or worsening heart failure before death.[65] †Multinational, mixed aetiology.[66]
*AIRE = Acute Infarction Ramipril Efficacy; †ATLAS = Assessment of Treatment with Lisinopril and Survival; HF = heart failure.

Multidisciplinary care for heart failure: the unmet need

I'm just a blood leech and monitor

General practitioner of Mr T, aged 69

Heart failure is a complex syndrome, and many non-specialist doctors feel uneasy about dealing with it, especially in the advanced stages. Nevertheless, the vast majority of heart failure is dealt with by non-specialists – general practitioners, junior hospital doctors and consultants in medical specialties other than cardiology. Even among cardiologists, there are many whose special interests do not extend to the management of end-stage disease. This is a strikingly different situation from that in cancer care, where every patient is likely to receive prompt care from a range of specialists. A palliative care professional who becomes involved in the management of a cancer patient can usually be certain that the diagnosis has been clearly established and that every curative or life-prolonging intervention has been tried or at least considered.

Although this cannot yet be claimed for heart failure, this situation is changing. In the UK, the National Service Framework for Coronary Heart Disease[67] in 2000 laid down a basic set of requirements for the care of patients with heart failure, including the involvement of palliative care and a timetable for progress. This was further set out in a National Institute for Clinical Excellence guideline for England and Wales in 2003, updated in 2010,[68] including the need for palliative care for people with moderate-to-severe heart failure.

A great step forward has come with the deployment of heart failure nurse specialists throughout the UK. Gradually, we are seeing the coming together of the necessary elements of a heart failure team in many parts of the country (*see* Table 1.5).

The role of palliative care services

The palliative care needs of people with heart failure are wide ranging and require a team approach to care. In this context, what is the appropriate role of SPC services and to what extent are they willing and able to be involved?

The survey of adult SPC services in England undertaken by Gibbs and colleagues[69] late in 2004 had a 60% response rate, with only three out of 222 respondents saying that they did not think SPC services had a role to play in end-stage heart failure. Around 60% of SPC services were already offering inpatient, day hospice and home care to such patients, albeit in small numbers only. The 2012–13 minimum dataset report from the National Council for Palliative Care in the UK showed that the proportion of patients accessing SPC services had increased, especially over the past 6–7 years. This was most pronounced in hospital liaison services, in which patients with a non-cancer diagnosis accounted for 27% of new referrals.[70]

Two national surveys of heart failure nurse specialists in England in 2005 and 2010 showed that the vast and increasing majority felt that they had a role in providing palliative care to their patients and that access to SPC services was important.[71] The role of specialist palliative care is discussed in more detail in Chapter 10.

TABLE 1.5 The heart failure team

Level of care	Team members	Sources of advice/education
Day-to-day care	• General practitioner • Practice nurse • District nurse	• Primary care training courses and study days • Written and online materials • Advice from heart failure specialist nurse, cardiologist
Regular back-up care	• Heart failure specialist nurse, community palliative care nurse, social services, heart failure clinic (community or hospital based), cardiac rehabilitation, community pharmacist • Occupational therapist • Physiotherapist	• Accredited courses for heart failure • Written and online materials • Specialist courses and conferences
Specialist services	• Cardiologist • Geriatrician • Palliative care physician • Chaplain • Clinical psychologist	• Written materials, online materials, specialist journals • Specialist courses and conferences • Tertiary referral, e.g. to cardiac surgeon, interventional cardiologist

PART 3: THE EVIDENCE BASE FOR THE PALLIATIVE CARE MANAGEMENT OF PATIENTS WITH HEART FAILURE

A summary of the empirical literature relating to palliative care interventions for heart failure allows us to comment on and evaluate the evidence base for palliative care management in heart failure. The interventions described in this section aimed to promote a palliative approach to care, provided by a range of multidisciplinary care providers and across a range of settings, and addressed multiple domains including physical, psychological and communication needs. Most were community-based approaches to integrating palliative care into the case management of patients with heart failure, such as the PhoenixCare home-based palliative care programme delivered by nurse case managers in the USA[72] and a heart failure palliative care specialist nurse model from the UK.[73] Community-based palliative care interventions seem particularly appropriate for patients with chronic conditions of unpredictable trajectory such as heart failure, as they can be feasibly integrated into the chronic care of patients. Indeed, a 2012 prospective observational study of integrated cardiology–palliative care teams in the UK reported that heart failure specialist nurses (HFSNs) were central to communicating and coordinating all aspects of end-of-life care.[74] However, the integration of palliative care into chronic disease management may present challenges for front-line staff, predominantly nurses. For example, an observational study in Scotland concluded that while some HFSNs could successfully integrate a palliative care approach effectively into the existing HFSN role, others found it to be more difficult due to the extra time required to perform the role and the additional education and training requirements.[75] Nonetheless, community-based interventions have been shown to improve the appropriateness, timeliness and continuity of patient care[73] and improve patient outcomes such as self-management of illness and symptom distress.[72]

Palliative care interventions such as goals-of-care and decision-making aids for patients with heart failure or chronic kidney disease and their caregivers have been evaluated in a randomised controlled trial, which demonstrated positive outcomes such as improved caregiver understanding of patient preferences.[76] However, interventions developed in the context of other conditions, notably cancer, have been less successful in demonstrating positive outcomes. For example, a randomised controlled trial exploring the impact of a psychosocial caregiver intervention (the 'COPE' intervention) on caregiver outcomes was unable to demonstrate any positive findings, despite the intervention having demonstrated positive outcomes in cancer.[77] This finding indicates a need for disease-specific interventions for patients with heart failure and their caregivers and suggests that generic approaches, or those developed for cancer, may not necessarily be appropriate without significant modification.

Palliative care programmes based in the outpatient setting have also been described in studies conducted in the USA and have successfully addressed issues including advanced care planning, care coordination and psychosocial issues.[78,79] Many of the issues addressed in these programmes are predicated on the belief that palliative heart failure care should be complementary to standard heart failure care at all stages of the disease process.[80] This issue was more explicitly addressed in a retrospective pilot study[81] to explore the clinical impact of palliative care involvement in patients referred for transplantation. Patients receiving SPC involvement had improved symptom control, improved satisfaction and more focused goals of care.

The evidence for the use of advance care planning (ACP) interventions in heart failure is, in the main, encouraging, with evidence of improved patient and surrogate outcomes for patients receiving ACP. Kirchhoff and colleagues[76,82] explored the impact of patient-centred advanced care planning (PC-ACP) in people with heart or renal failure on the achievement of patient preferences and surrogate understanding of disease, using a randomised controlled trial design. They reported that PC-ACP resulted in more patients' wishes being met with regard to cardiopulmonary resuscitation and that surrogates of PC-ACP patients had better understanding of patient goals than surrogates of controls. Preliminary data from the implementation of ACP tools, such as disease-specific advance care planning, are promising, showing increased hospice use and more documented directives in participants than those who did not use the tools.[83] However, as with the use of ACP in other conditions such as chronic obstructive pulmonary disease,[84] barriers – including physician engagement with ACP and inconsistent method of referral – have hampered efforts to fully integrate ACP into the care of patients with end-stage heart failure.[85]

While palliative care interventions are now widely used among patients with heart failure, evidence from randomised controlled trials regarding the effectiveness of these interventions is relatively limited. One trial of house-bound terminally ill patients (35% with heart failure), compared usual care with a community-based, multidisciplinary-team, palliative care intervention plus usual care.[86] Participants in the palliative care arm experienced significantly increased patient satisfaction, reduced use of medical services and healthcare costs, and were more likely to die at home than in hospital. Several randomised controlled trials of palliative care interventions in heart failure are ongoing, and recent pilot data published from the Palliative advanced home caRE and heart FailurE caRe (PREFER) trial are encouraging.[87] Trial evidence for palliative care interventions with heart failure patients tailored to the unique characteristics of their condition are needed, as careful consideration should be given to the specific issues facing this group of patients. Well-known palliative care interventions, such as ACP, have now been widely used in heart failure and evidence is mounting for their effectiveness. However, there is some way to go before engagement with clinical staff is achieved across all settings. Approaches that advocate the integration of SPC services with chronic care or even curative care are becoming increasingly popular, reflecting an increasing recognition that palliative care in heart failure should become a core component of a fully integrated approach to care.

REFERENCES

1 Hinton JM. The physical and mental distress of the dying. *Q J Med.* 1963; **32**: 1–21.

2 Barnes S, Gott M, Payne S *et al.* Prevalence of symptoms in a community-based sample of heart failure patients. *J Pain Symptom Manage.* 2006; **32**(3): 208–16.

3 Friedman MM. Older adults' symptoms and their duration before hospitalization for heart failure. *Heart Lung.* 1997; **26**(3): 169–76.

4 Evangelista LS, Dracup K, Doering LV. Treatment-seeking delays in heart failure patients. *J Heart Lung Transplant.* 2000; **19**(10): 932–8.

5 Barnes S, Gott M, Payne S *et al.* Recruiting older people into a large, community-based study of heart failure. *Chronic Illn.* 2005; **1**(4): 321–9.

6 Austin J, Williams WR, Hutchison S. Patterns of fatigue in elderly heart failure patients measured by a quality of life scale (Minnesota living with heart failure). *Eur J Cardiovasc Nurs.* 2012; **11**(4): 439–44.

7 Goldberg RJ, Spencer FA, Szklo-Coxe M *et al.* Symptom presentation in patients hospitalized with acute heart failure. *Clin Cardiol.* 2010; **33**(6):E73–80.

8 Aldred H, Gott M, Gariballa S. Advanced heart failure: impact on older patients and informal carers. *J Adv Nurs.* 2005; **49**(2): 116–24.

9 Yohannes AM, Willgoss TG, Baldwin RC *et al.* Depression and anxiety in chronic heart failure and chronic obstructive pulmonary disease: prevalence, relevance, clinical implications and management principles. *Int J Geriatr Psychiatry.* 2010; **25**(12): 1209–21.

10 Turvey CL, Schultz K, Arndt S *et al.* Prevalence and correlates of depressive symptoms in a community sample of people suffering from heart failure. *J Am Geriatr Soc.* 2002; **50**(12): 2003–8.

11 Hobbs FD, Kenkre JE, Roalfe AK *et al.* Impact of heart failure and left ventricular systolic dysfunction on quality of life: a cross-sectional study comparing common chronic cardiac and medical disorders and a representative adult population. *Eur Heart J.* 2002; **23**(23): 1867–76.

12 Levenson JW, McCarthy EP, Lynn J *et al.* The last six months of life for patients with congestive heart failure. *J Am Geriatr Soc.* 2000; **48**(5 Suppl.):S101–9.

13 Nordgren L, Sorensen S. Symptoms experienced in the last six months of life in patients with end-stage heart failure. *Eur J Cardiovasc Nurs.* 2003; **2**(3): 213–17.

14 Rogers A, Addington-Hall JM, McCoy AS *et al.* A qualitative study of chronic heart failure patients' understanding of their symptoms and drug therapy. *Eur J Heart Fail.* 2002; **4**(3): 283–7.

15 Small N, Barnes S, Gott M *et al.* Dying, death and bereavement: a qualitative study of the views of carers of people with heart failure in the UK. *BMC Palliat Care.* 2009; **8**: 6.

16 Barclay S, Momen N, Case-Upton S *et al.* End-of-life care conversations with heart failure patients: a systematic literature review and narrative synthesis. *Br J Gen Pract.* 2011; **61**(582):e49–62.

17 Waterworth S, Gott M. Decision making among older people with advanced heart failure as they transition to dependency and death. *Curr Opin Support Palliat Care.* 2010; **4**(4): 238–42.

18 Clark D. Between hope and acceptance: the medicalisation of dying. *BMJ.* 2002; **324**(7342): 905–7.

19 Gott M, Small N, Barnes S *et al.* Older people's views of a good death in heart failure: implications for palliative care provision. *Soc Sci Med.* 2008; **67**(7): 1113–21.

20 Davis MP, Albert NM, Young JB. Palliation of heart failure. *Am J Hosp Palliat Care.* 2005; **22**(3): 211–22.

21 Goodlin SJ. Palliative care in congestive heart failure. *J Am Coll Cardiol.* 2009; **54**(5): 386–96.

22 Lunney JR, Lynn J, Foley DJ *et al.* Patterns of functional decline at the end of life. *JAMA.* 2003; **289**(18): 2387–92.

23 Gott M, Barnes S, Parker C *et al.* Dying trajectories in heart failure. *Palliat Med.* 2007; **21**(2): 95–9.

24 Hauptman PJ, Havranek EP. Integrating palliative care into heart failure care. *Arch Intern Med.* 2005; **165**(4): 374–8.

25 Johnson MJ, Gadoud A. Palliative care for people with chronic heart failure: when is it time? *J Palliat Care.* 2011; **27**(1): 37–42.

26 Jerant AF, Azari RS, Nesbitt TS *et al.* The TLC model of palliative care in the elderly: preliminary application in the assisted living setting. *Ann Fam Med.* 2004; **2**(1): 54–60.

27 Gadoud A, Kane E, Macleod U *et al.* Palliative care among heart failure patients in primary care: a comparison to cancer patients using English family practice data. *PLoS One.* 2014; **9**(11): e113188.

28 Davidson PM. Difficult conversations and chronic heart failure: do you talk the talk or walk the walk? *Curr Opin Support Palliat Care.* 2007; **1**(4): 274–8.

29 O'Leary N, Murphy NF, O'Loughlin C *et al.* A comparative study of the palliative care needs of heart failure and cancer patients. *Eur J Heart Fail.* 2009; **11**(4): 406–12.

30 Green E, Gardiner C, Gott M *et al.* Exploring the extent of communication surrounding transitions to palliative care in heart failure: the perspectives of health care professionals. *J Palliat Care.* 2011; **27**(2): 107–16.

31 General Medical Council (GMC). *Treatment and Care Towards the End of Life: good practice in decision-making.* London: GMC; 2010. Available at: www.gmc-uk.org/Treatment_and_care_towards_the_end_of_life___English_0914.pdf_48902105.pdf (accessed 7 May 2015).

32 O'Callaghan A, Laking G, Frey R *et al.* Can we predict which hospitalised patients are in their last year of life? A prospective cross-sectional study of the Gold Standards Framework Prognostic Indicator Guidance as a screening tool in the acute hospital setting. *Palliat Med.* 2014; **28**(8): 1046–52.

33 Haga K, Murray S, Reid J *et al.* Identifying community based chronic heart failure patients in the last year of life: a comparison of the Gold Standards Framework Prognostic Indicator Guide and the Seattle Heart Failure Model. *Heart.* 2012; **98**(7): 579–83.

34 Fenning SJ. Why identify 'end-of-life' in palliative care? *BMJ Support Palliat Care.* 2014; **4**(1): 6.

35 Boyd K, Murray SA. Recognising and managing key transitions in end of life care. *BMJ.* 2010; **341**: c4863.

36 Waller A, Girgis A, Davidson PM *et al.* Facilitating needs-based support and palliative care for people with chronic heart failure: preliminary evidence for the acceptability, inter-rater reliability, and validity of a needs assessment tool. *J Pain Symptom Manage.* 2012; **45**(5): 912–25.

37 Jaarsma T, Beattie JM, Ryder M *et al.* Palliative care in heart failure: a position state-ment from the palliative care workshop of the Heart Failure Association of the European Society of Cardiology. *Eur J Heart Fail.* 2009; 11(5): 433–43.

38 Anderson H, Ward C, Eardley A *et al.* The concerns of patients under palliative care and a heart failure clinic are not being met. *Palliat Med.* 2001; 15(4): 279–86.

39 Molloy GJ, Johnston DW, Witham MD. Family caregiving and congestive heart fail-ure. Review and analysis. *Eur J Heart Fail.* 2005; 7(4): 592–603.

40 McKinley RK, Stokes T, Exley C *et al.* Care of people dying with malignant and cardi-orespiratory disease in general practice. *Br J Gen Pract.* 2004; 54(509): 909–13.

41 Levenson JW, McCarthy EP, Lynn J *et al.* Symptoms experienced in the last six months of life with end-stage heart failure. *J Am Geriatr Soc.* 2000; 48(5 Suppl.): S101–9.

42 Ng K, von Gunten CF. Symptoms and attitudes of 100 consecutive patients admit-ted to an acute hospice/palliative care unit. *J Pain Symptom Manage.* 1998; 16(5): 307–16.

43 Pantilat SZ, O'Riordan DL, Dibble SL *et al.* Longitudinal assessment of symptom severity among hospitalized elders diagnosed with cancer, heart failure, and chronic obstructive pulmonary disease. *J Hosp Med.* 2012; 7(7): 567–72.

44 Solano JP, Gomes B, Higginson IJ. A comparison of symptom prevalence in far advanced cancer, AIDS, heart disease, chronic obstructive pulmonary disease and renal disease. *J Pain Symptom Manage.* 2006; 31(1): 58–69.

45 Murray SA, Boyd K, Kendall M *et al.* Dying of lung cancer or cardiac failure: prospec-tive qualitative interview study of patients and their carers in the community. *BMJ.* 2002; 325(7370): 929.

46 Rogers A, Karlsen S, Addington-Hall JM. Dying for care: the experiences of terminally ill cancer patients in hospital in an inner city health district. *Palliat Med.* 2000; 14(1): 53–4.

47 Rogers AE, Addington-Hall JM, Abery AJ *et al.* Knowledge and communication diffi-culties for patients with chronic heart failure: qualitative study. *BMJ.* 2000; 321(7261): 605–7.

48 Stewart S, Macintyre K, Hole DJ *et al.* More 'malignant' than cancer? Five-year survival following a first admission for heart failure. *Eur J Heart Fail.* 2001; 3(3): 315–22.

49 Cowie MR, Wood DA, Coats AJ *et al.* Survival of patients with a new diagnosis of heart failure: a population based study. *Heart.* 2000; 83(5): 505–10.

50 Braunschweig F, Cowie MR, Auricchio A. What are the costs of heart failure? *Europace.* 2011; 13 Suppl. 2: ii13–17.

51 Martínez-Sellés M, Doughty RN, Poppe K *et al.* Gender and survival in patients with heart failure: interactions with diabetes and aetiology. Results from the MAGGIC individual patient meta-analysis. *Eur J Heart Fail.* 2012; 14(5): 473–9.

52 Mercer BN, Morais S, Cubbon RM *et al.* Diabetes mellitus and the heart. *Int J Clin Pract.* 2012; 66(7): 640–7.

53 Braunstein JB, Anderson GF, Gerstenblith G *et al.* Noncardiac comorbidity increases preventable hospitalizations and mortality among Medicare beneficiaries with chronic heart failure. *J Am Coll Cardiol.* 2003; 42(7): 1226–33.

54 Hanratty B, Hibbert D, Mair F *et al.* Doctors' perceptions of palliative care for heart failure: focus group study. *BMJ.* 2002; 325(7364): 581–5.

55 Beattie JM, Murray RG, Brittle J *et al.* Palliative care in terminal cardiac failure. Small

numbers of patients with terminal cardiac failure may make considerable demands on services. *BMJ.* 1995; **310**(6991): 1411.

56 Gannon C. Palliative care in terminal cardiac failure. Hospices cannot fulfil such a vast and diverse role. *BMJ.* 1995; **310**(6991): 1410–11.

57 Mosterd A, Hoes AW. Clinical epidemiology of heart failure. *Heart.* 2007; **93**(9): 1137–46.

58 Unal B, Critchley JA, Capewell S. Missing, mediocre, or merely obsolete? An evaluation of UK data sources for coronary heart disease. *J Epidemiol Community Health.* 2003; **57**(7): 530–5.

59 Blackledge HM, Tomlinson J, Squire IB. Prognosis for patients newly admitted to hospital with heart failure: survival trends in 12 220 index admissions in Leicestershire 1993–2001. *Heart.* 2003; **89**(6): 615–20.

60 Sosin MD, Bhatia GS, Davis RC *et al.* Heart failure – the importance of ethnicity. *Eur J Heart Fail.* 2004; **6**(7): 831–43.

61 Newton JD, Blackledge HM, Squire IB. Ethnicity and variation in prognosis for patients newly hospitalised for heart failure: a matched historical cohort study. *Heart.* 2005; **91**(12): 1545–50.

62 Sosin MD, Bhatia GS, Zarifis J *et al.* An 8-year follow-up study of acute admissions with heart failure in a multiethnic population. *Eur J Heart Fail.* 2004; **6**(5): 669–72.

63 Galasko GI, Senior R, Lahiri A. Ethnic differences in the prevalence and aetiology of left ventricular systolic dysfunction in the community: the Harrow heart failure watch. *Heart.* 2005; **91**(5): 595–600.

64 Blackledge HM, Newton J, Squire IB. Prognosis for South Asian and white patients newly admitted to hospital with heart failure in the United Kingdom: historical cohort study. *BMJ.* 2003; **327**(7414): 526–31.

65 Cleland JG, Erhardt L, Murray G *et al.* Effect of ramipril on morbidity and mode of death among survivors of acute myocardial infarction with clinical evidence of heart failure. A report from the AIRE Study Investigators. *Eur Heart J.* 1997; **18**(1): 41–51.

66 Poole-Wilson PA, Uretsky BF, Thygesen K *et al.* Mode of death in heart failure: findings from the ATLAS trial. *Heart.* 2003; **89**(1): 42–8.

67 Department of Health. *National Service Framework for Coronary Heart Disease: modern standards and service models.* London: Department of Health; 2000. Available at: www.gov.uk/government/uploads/system/uploads/attachment_data/file/198931/ National_Service_Framework_for_Coronary_Heart_Disease.pdf (accessed 8 May 2015).

68 National Institute for Health and Clinical Excellence. *Chronic Heart Failure: management of chronic heart failure in adults in primary and secondary care.* NICE guideline CG108. London: National Institute for Health and Clinical Excellence; 2010. www.nice.org.uk/guidance/CG108

69 Gibbs LM, Khatri AK, Gibbs JS. Survey of specialist palliative care and heart failure: September 2004. *Palliat Med.* 2006; **20**(6): 603–9.

70 National Council for Palliative Care. *National Survey of Patient Activity Data for Specialist Palliative Care Services: MDS full report for the year 2011–2012.* London: National Council for Palliative Care; 2012. Available at: www.ncpc.org.uk/sites/ default/files/MDS%20Full%20Report%202012.pdf (accessed 5 July 2014).

71 Johnson MJ, MacCallum A, Butler J *et al.* Heart failure specialist nurses' use of

palliative care services: a comparison of surveys across England in 2005 and 2010. *Eur J Cardiovasc Nurs*. 2011; **11**(2): 190–6.

72 Aiken LS, Butner J, Lockhart CA *et al*. Outcome evaluation of a randomized trial of the PhoenixCare intervention: program of case management and coordinated care for the seriously chronically ill. *J Palliat Med*. 2006; **9**(1): 111–26.

73 Rogers A. *Role of the British Heart Foundation Heart Failure Palliative Care Specialist Nurse*. London: British Heart Foundation; 2010. Available at: www.bhf.org.uk/~/media/files/publications/about-the-bhf/z812_role_of_the_bhf_heart_failure_palliative_care_specialist_nurse_a_retrospective_evaluation_0111.pdf (accessed 8 May 2015).

74 Johnson M, Nunn A, Hawkes T *et al*. Planning for end of life care in people with heart failure: experience of two integrated cardiology-palliative care teams. *Br J Cardiol*. 2012; **19**(2): 71–5.

75 Millerick Y, Wright J, Freeman A. *British Heart Foundation Heart Failure Palliative Care Project Report: the Glasgow and Clyde experience*. Final report. London: British Heart Foundation; 2010. Available at: www.bhf.org.uk/~/media/files/publications/about-the-bhf/z811_bhf_heart_failure_palliative_care_project_report_the_glasgow_and_clyde_experience_0111.pdf (accessed 8 May 2015).

76 Kirchhoff KT, Hammes BJ, Kehl KA *et al*. Effect of a disease-specific planning intervention on surrogate understanding of patient goals for future medical treatment. *J Am Geriatr Soc*. 2010; **58**(7): 1233–40.

77 McMillan SC, Small BJ, Haley WE *et al*. The COPE intervention for caregivers of patients with heart failure: an adapted intervention. *J Hosp Palliat Nurs*. 2013; **15**(4). doi:10.1097/NJH.06013e31827777fb.

78 Bekelman DB, Nowels CT, Allen LA *et al*. Outpatient palliative care for chronic heart failure: a case series. *J Palliat Med*. 2011; **14**(7): 815–21.

79 Evangelista LS, Lombardo D, Malik S *et al*. Examining the effects of an outpatient palliative care consultation on symptom burden, depression, and quality of life in patients with symptomatic heart failure. *J Card Fail*. 2012; **18**(12): 894–9.

80 Bekelman DB, Nowels CT, Retrum JH *et al*. Giving voice to patients' and family caregivers' needs in chronic heart failure: implications for palliative care programs. *J Palliat Med*. 2011; **14**(12): 1317–24.

81 Schwarz ER, Baraghoush A, Morrissey RP *et al*. Pilot study of palliative care consultation in patients with advanced heart failure referred for cardiac transplantation. *J Palliat Med*. 2012; **15**(1): 12–15.

82 Kirchhoff KT, Hammes BJ, Kehl KA *et al*. Effect of a disease-specific advance care planning intervention on end-of-life care. *J Am Geriatr Soc*. 2012; **60**(5): 946–50.

83 Schellinger S, Sidebottom A, Briggs L. Disease specific advance care planning for heart failure patients: implementation in a large health system. *J Palliat Med*. 2011; **14**(11): 1224–30.

84 Gott M, Gardiner C, Small N *et al*. Barriers to advance care planning in chronic obstructive pulmonary disease. *Palliat Med*. 2009; **23**(7): 642–8.

85 Ahluwalia SC, Levin JR, Lorenz KA *et al*. 'There's no cure for this condition': how physicians discuss advance care planning in heart failure. *Patient Educ Couns*. 2013; **91**(2): 200–5.

86 Brumley R, Enguidanos S, Jamison P *et al*. Increased satisfaction with care and lower

costs: results of a randomized trial of in-home palliative care. *J Am Geriatr Soc*. 2007; 55(7): 993–1000.

87 Brannstrom M, Boman K. Effects of person-centred and integrated chronic heart failure and palliative home care. PREFER: a randomized controlled study. *Eur J Heart Fail*. 2014; 16(10): 1142–51.

CHAPTER 2

The syndrome of advanced heart failure

RICHARD LEHMAN AND SHONA JENKINS

INTRODUCTION

Heart failure often begins insidiously, but its end-stage is a lethal syndrome that affects every organ and system in the body. Despite all the advances in treatment of the past two decades, heart failure kills because it sets in train a number of physiological and chemical responses that combine into a downward spiral.[1] On top of this, episodes of infection, inappropriate treatment or electrical instability can lead to 'decompensation', and, at all stages of heart failure, there is a risk of sudden death from electrical instability or new infarction. This chapter attempts to summarise the processes of advanced heart failure for the non-specialist reader to explain why heart failure tends to get worse and why it produces its wide range of symptoms.

AETIOLOGY

In most Western countries, around two-thirds of heart failure can be attributed to ischaemic heart disease. Other common causes are hypertension, valvular heart disease, adult congenital heart disease and various cardiomyopathies (e.g. familial, alcohol related or secondary to cytotoxic drugs or obesity). People with heart failure may have left ventricular dysfunction (heart failure with reduced ejection fraction [HFrEF]) or preserved ejection fraction (heart failure with preserved ejection fraction) but with other structural and functional cardiac abnormalities. Major contributors to heart failure with preserved ejection fraction are ageing, hypertension and diabetes mellitus, and morbidity and mortality rival those of HFrEF although the underlying pathophysiology is less well understood.[2] The following discussion refers primarily to HFrEF. As we saw in Chapter 1, 'The need for palliative care in heart failure', the epidemiology of heart failure is a vexed subject, due to differences of definition, but these need not concern us here. All these processes eventually lead to the same syndrome in the final stage.

The age distribution of heart failure is presented in Figure 2.1. The vast majority of heart failure patients are aged over 65 years old and increasingly liable to other age-related problems.

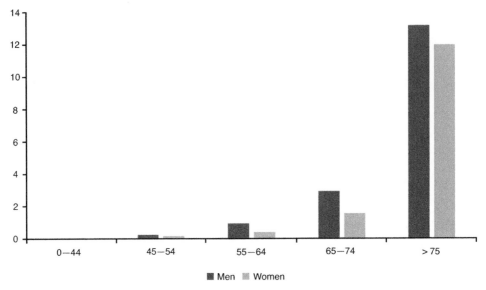

FIGURE 2.1 Prevalence of heart failure in UK by age and sex 2011
Source: Adapted from British Heart Foundation statistics.[3]

THE FAILING PUMP

The traditional model of heart failure simply looked at the heart as a pump and heart failure as a mechanical process due to impaired pumping. The key factors were seen as:

- strength of contraction
- the amount of fluid in the circulation (preload)
- peripheral resistance (afterload).

Heart muscle cells are so designed that the more they are stretched, the harder they contract – this is known as 'Starling's law'. However, when the limit is reached, ventricular failure ensues. Failure of the right ventricle means that the systemic venous circulation cannot be cleared properly, so that peripheral venous pressure rises. This results in:

- visibly elevated jugular venous pressure
- liver congestion
- peripheral oedema.

Failure of the left ventricle means that the venous circulation of the lungs cannot be cleared properly, so that the pulmonary venous pressure rises. This results in:

- breathlessness (dyspnoea)
- breathlessness when lying down (orthopnoea)
- audible crackles at the lung bases.

This takes us a certain distance in understanding the symptoms of heart failure and the logic of its therapy. Historically, both preload and afterload were reduced by bleeding or leeches in addition to fluid and salt restriction. Contemporary heart failure management now comprises diuretics to expel sodium and water, which is given alongside angiotensin-converting enzyme (ACE) inhibitors, beta-blockers and mineralocorticoid receptor antagonists. These drugs variably reduce preload and afterload, in addition to counteracting the deleterious effects of inappropriate neurohumoral activation in heart failure (*see* section RAAS and Chapter 3, 'Optimal therapy for heart failure').

Using this model, it would also seem logical to use drugs that increase the contractile strength of heart muscle, known as 'inotropes'. Such drugs are still widely used in the management of acute heart failure in hospital settings, but their long-term use is always associated with increases in mortality, for reasons that will become clearer shortly.[4]

This relatively simple model of heart failure is still a useful starting point, but it fails to explain many of the features of heart failure as a progressive syndrome. For this, we need to look in greater depth at what happens to the heart itself and with greater breadth at the effects that this has on the rest of the body.

CELL DEATH

The basis of the heart's pumping action is a collection of specialised muscle cells known collectively as the 'myocardium', and individually as 'cardiac myocytes'. Their number, like the number of brain cells, is effectively fixed early in life, so that when they die, they are not replaced. In fact this is not strictly true for either heart or brain cells, but in both organs, unlike in many others such as the liver or the skin, there is no effective repair mechanism to replace dead cells. The remaining cells need to work harder. We have seen that myocytes are designed to beat harder the more they are stretched. This stretching process triggers a number of cellular mechanisms, which include the release of hormones (A- and B-type natriuretic peptides) to try to relieve preload, and an increase in myosin, which leads to the cells individually becoming bigger and stronger. This is called 'hypertrophy', and it results in an increase in thickness of the ventricular wall – not because there are more cells, but because the cells are bigger. These adaptive mechanisms are very effective in allowing myocytes to cope with a wide range of extra demands. Myocytes can die by two mechanisms, known by the Greek terms 'necrosis' and 'apoptosis'.[5] 'Necrosis' directly means 'turning into a corpse', referring to sudden, disorganised cell death. 'Apoptosis' is a modern coinage meaning something like 'curling up', a programmed and orderly kind of cell death.

Necrosis of heart muscle is a common and often dramatic event witnessed every day in acute general hospitals. It is caused by the sudden occlusion of a coronary artery, leading to loss of blood supply to a segment of ventricle, usually the left. The tissue death that results is known as 'infarction', and it consists of the mass necrosis of cells deprived of oxygen and nutrients. Necrotic myocytes burst and release their cell contents, leading to electrical instability and the risk of sudden death from ventricular fibrillation. The infarcted segment of ventricle becomes mechanically unstable, leading to ventricular wall weakness or even rupture. If the patient survives, the necrotic area heals by a process of mass fibrosis, which can impair its blood supply further.

Apoptosis is the process of cells deciding that enough is enough. Many cells in the body are programmed to make this decision within days or weeks, and are duly replaced by similar cells. However, cardiac myocytes are programmed to use apoptosis as the last resort, when they have been overstretched or undernourished for years or decades. The commonest reasons are long-standing hypertension leading to chronic pathological hypertrophy, or diffuse ischaemia; diabetes is often associated with both these processes. The process of apoptosis is orderly and does not cause the release of toxins or immediate electrical or mechanical instability. However, the lost myocytes are replaced only by fibrous tissue, meaning that the remaining myocytes have to work harder and may 'decide' on apoptosis sooner. In this way, the failing heart becomes progressively depleted of working cells.

REMODELLING

Death of heart muscle, especially by necrosis, is followed by a process of reshaping the muscles of the entire ventricle in response to the changed distribution of mechanical load. This is called 'remodelling', and it can either be favourable or unfavourable (adverse) for the future of the heart.[6] Favourable remodelling is a process of 'tightening up', so that the ventricle regains the size and shape that allow efficient pumping. Adverse remodelling is a process in which the damaged ventricle becomes progressively stretched. When the word 'remodelling' is used on its own in the heart failure literature, it usually refers to adverse remodelling. This can be symmetrical, leading to a bigger, floppier ventricle, in which the myocytes are continuously overstretched and therefore likely to die off gradually by apoptosis. Even worse, it can be asymmetrical, in which there is a weak, bulging aneurysmal area of ventricular wall due to a large area of infarction. As well as making ventricular contraction less efficient, and predisposing to the formation of ventricular thrombus, this stresses the adjacent muscle segments and carries an additional risk of electrical instability.

THE RENIN–ANGIOTENSIN–ALDOSTERONE SYSTEM (RAAS)

This system of hormones is designed to preserve blood flow to the kidneys in the event of sudden haemorrhage, or some other other problem leading to a drop in BP or circulating volume. Therefore, it is designed to work rapidly to raise blood pressure and retain sodium and water. In other words, it is there to increase preload and keep it increased. Heart failure acts as a trigger to activate the RAAS, because the failing heart sends less blood to the kidneys. This sets up a vicious cycle in which the RAAS increases preload and further overburdens the heart.

The RAAS has been the main target for therapeutic innovation in heart failure over the past 20 years, so that we can now potentially block every stage of the cascade (*see* Figure 2.2). However, this is a therapeutic strategy with diminishing returns and carries with it the danger of hyperkalaemia and hypotension

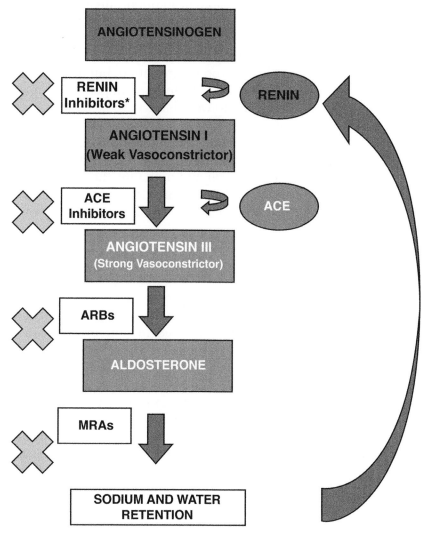

FIGURE 2.2 The renin–angiotensin–aldosterone system

Note: *Renin inhibitors are not yet licensed in heart failure.

ACE = angiotensin-converting enzyme; ARBs = angiotensin receptor blockers; MRAs = mineralocorticoid receptor antagonists.

if carried too far. Most patients with systolic heart failure should be on some form of RAAS-blocking medication, but how much and how many kinds are issues that remain contentious (*see* Chapter 3).

SYMPATHETIC NERVOUS SYSTEM

The sympathetic nervous system governs the rate of the heart either by adrenaline and noradrenaline released into the circulation, mainly from the adrenal glands, or by direct adrenergic innervation to the atrium. Once again, falling output from the failing heart triggers a response aimed at elevating blood pressure to maintain essential organ perfusion. In addition, adrenergic stimulation increases the rate of the heart in an attempt to increase cardiac output, at the same time as increasing afterload by shutting down peripheral arterioles. Just as with RAAS activation, these are useful responses to sudden blood loss or other emergencies involving a temporary drop in circulation, but they are harmful to the failing heart in a number of ways. An increase in peripheral resistance (afterload) means that the heart has to work harder. An increase in heart rate means that the filling of the ventricles and the coronary arteries is less efficient. Up to a decade ago, adrenergic stimulant drugs were being used in heart failure to increase cardiac output and improve symptoms. When it became clear that they actually increased progression and mortality, the opposite strategy was tried, and now cardio-selective beta-adrenergic blocking drugs are used in all classes of heart failure with benefits at least as great as those of RAAS-blocking drugs.

CARDIAC PERFUSION

Contracting myocytes need a good oxygen supply. Another vicious cycle can come about because the oxygen supply to the heart is partly dependent on the heart's own function. If there is pulmonary oedema, the oxygenation of the blood is impaired. If the heart is beating too fast, then the coronary arteries do not have time to fill properly during diastole. These factors are worsened by narrowing of the coronary arteries by atheroma and distortion of the coronary microvasculature by myocardial fibrosis. The result may be that parts of the ventricle go into a state of paralysis known as 'hibernation'. The myocytes are alive but inactive and can be restored to full function by improving the delivery of oxygen to them. This is the rationale for attempting coronary reperfusion (by percutaneous procedures or by coronary artery bypass grafting) in heart failure. However, whether this strategy confers morbidity or mortality benefit remains contentious.[7]

DECOMPENSATION: WHEN CHRONIC BECOMES ACUTE

In acute heart failure (decompensation), all the mechanisms that we have discussed come into play in a catastrophic sequence. Extra demand on the heart as a result of the factors listed following leads to sympathetic activation, which speeds the heart rate. This leads to impaired filling of the ventricles and the coronary arteries, producing a fall in cardiac output and a degree of ischaemic stress on the already compromised heart. The RAAS also comes into action, adding to the fluid load. Pulmonary oedema builds rapidly and further impairs oxygenation of the heart and the whole body. If the situation continues unchecked, the patient becomes cyanotic and intensely distressed, with pulmonary oedema. Intravenous diuretics and high-concentration oxygen are vital in this situation. The common precipitants of decompensation are:

- ischaemia or infarction
- arrhythmia
- anaemia
- inappropriate drug treatment – for example, non-steroidal anti-inflammatory drugs, glitazones
- inappropriate cessation of drug treatment – for instance, non-compliance
- metabolic disorders such as hyperthyroidism or uncontrolled diabetes.

RHYTHM AND SYNCHRONY

The proportion of heart failure patients with atrial fibrillation rises from less than 10% in New York Heart Association (NYHA) class I to approximately 50% in NYHA class IV.[8] This arrhythmia greatly impairs the heart's ability to respond to changes in demand. Thus, the onset of atrial fibrillation in an already impaired heart may lead to the cycle of decompensation just described. While electrical instability of the atrium is undesirable, electrical instability of the ventricle is immediately life threatening. Episodes of ventricular tachycardia can lead to fatal ventricular fibrillation, and the best way to prevent this is by implanting a cardiac defibrillator device (implantable cardiovertor defibrillator, or 'ICD'). This technology is expensive and raises difficult issues at the end of life, as discussed in Chapter 3 and Chapter 8 ('Care of the patient dying from heart failure'). As many as a third of heart failure patients also have impaired synchronisation between the two ventricles.[9] This can be corrected by a sophisticated pacing procedure known as 'cardiac resynchronisation therapy', or just 'biventricular pacing' (*see* Chapter 3, p. 51). This can improve life expectancy and quality of life.

SKELETAL MUSCLE AND CYTOKINES

The degree of functional impairment in heart failure is poorly related to systolic function but closely related to skeletal muscle function.[10] This varies greatly between individuals and is a subject of much ongoing research. Individuals with good skeletal muscle function can have minimal symptoms despite severe systolic impairment. Conversely, individuals with declining skeletal muscle function feel weak and breathless, lose muscle and become cachectic. They have a poor prognosis.[11] The determinants of these differences may be partly genetic and partly due to the release of cytokines. Cytokines are a large group of chemicals that feature in the process of inflammation, and their levels are usually raised in heart failure. Many cytokines are known to trigger wasting of skeletal muscle and apoptosis of heart muscle.[12] Struggling skeletal muscles stimulate respiratory effort and adrenergic output by means of ergo-reflexes. In heart failure, these reflexes are exaggerated, and this may be another vicious circle leading to increased demand on the weakening heart. Therapeutic approaches that have been tried are:

- blocking of cytokines; for example, tumour necrosis factor-alpha blockade with etanercept or infliximab. Unfortunately, trials showed increased mortality in heart failure and tumour necrosis factor-alpha-blocking drugs have now been shown to carry a danger of precipitating acute heart failure[13]
- muscle-training programmes: these have been shown to have some short-term functional benefit but no proven mortality benefit as yet.[14]

BREATHING

Breathlessness is a key feature of heart failure and forms part of the basis of the NYHA classification. Contributing factors are:
- pulmonary oedema – back pressure on the lung veins from an overloaded left atrium
- overdrive of the breathing muscles by chemoreceptors, which become over-sensitive to carbon-dioxide levels
- weakness of breathing muscles
- abnormal ventilatory patterns.

There are also characteristic changes in breathing patterns that are associated with heart failure:
- waking breathless in the night – paroxysmal nocturnal dyspnoea
- breathlessness on lying down – orthopnoea
- turning automatically to lie on the right side – trepopnoea[15]
- breathlessness on bending down – bendopnoea[16]
- long gaps in breathing – apnoeic breathing patterns, or Cheyne–Stokes breathing.

These breathing patterns also occur in other diseases, though trepopnoea is commonest in heart failure, and Cheyne–Stokes breathing by day is uncommon except in advanced heart failure.[17] In heart failure, these patterns are caused by a mixture of shifting pulmonary oedema and chemoreceptor overdrive. Continuous positive airway pressure may improve cardiac function, blood pressure, exercise capacity and quality of life for those with chronic heart failure and abnormal nocturnal breathing patterns, although evidence of benefit on survival is less clear.[18-21] There is some evidence that nocturnal continuous oxygen may be beneficial.[22]

NUTRITION AND ANAEMIA

Impaired appetite is common in heart failure and may be due to:

- congestion of the liver due to venous back-pressure
- oedema of the bowel, releasing 'feel-bad' toxins[23]
- depression.

Many non-obese patients with chronic heart failure may have an inadequate intake of calories and protein.[24] A good diet may be important in the avoidance of skeletal muscle loss and cachexia: this is an area of uncertainty and ongoing research.[25] Anaemia is very common in heart failure and is associated with poor outcomes.[26] The anaemia of advanced heart failure is not completely understood but contributing factors probably include malnutrition (iron, B11, B12), chronic blood loss, haemodilution, ACE-inhibitor therapy, bone-marrow malfunction and renal impairment.[27,28] One large randomised controlled trial demonstrated symptom improvement with intravenous iron in patients with NYHA class II–III heart failure and associated iron deficiency.[29] However, importantly, many of the patients in this study were not anaemic, with a mean haemoglobin at the start of the study of 11.9 g/dL. It was subsequently postulated that patients with heart failure and anaemia not due to iron deficiency would benefit from an erythropoietin-stimulating agent to increase haemoglobin. However, when this hypothesis was assessed in a randomised controlled trial, there was no clinical benefit and, in fact, an excess of thrombotic events in the darbepoetin group.[30]

DISTURBED SLEEP

Heart failure patients often sleep badly and wake unrefreshed.[31] This can be due to:

- breathing disturbances
- nocturia caused by diuretics and by disruption of the normal nightly pattern of antidiuretic hormone (or arginine vasopressin) secretion
- depression.

Poor sleep often adds an additional burden of daytime tiredness to the fatigue already experienced by most heart failure patients.

MOOD

There is an extensive literature on psychological factors in heart failure, which was reviewed in 2002[32] and 2005.[33] Many patients with heart failure are depressed, especially older people.[34] Depression is associated with a worse prognosis, interacting in a complex physical way with the disease mechanisms of heart failure.[35] Pathophysiological causes of depression in advanced heart failure include:

- cytokine release, which depletes brain stores of tryptophan and hence serotonin[36]

- possible direct effects from bacterial endotoxins leaking through oedematous bowel[37]
- possible direct effects from neuroendocrine activation (increased free adrenaline and noradrenaline)
- possible direct effects from periods of brain hypoxia.

Heart failure can also lead to depression for psychosocial reasons, because it is associated with:
- dependency
- weakness
- social isolation
- near-death episodes.

These issues need to be addressed in the holistic care of all heart failure patients. There may also be a place for some types of antidepressant drug treatment (*see* Chapter 6, 'Supportive care: psychological, social and spiritual aspects').

COGNITIVE DIFFICULTY

Many patients with heart failure experience difficulties in thinking, and heart failure is associated with a higher rate of cognitive decline and of brain-tissue loss.[38] This may be due to:
- coexisting cerebrovascular disease
- periods of cerebral hypoxia caused by Cheyne–Stokes breathing
- the effect of cytokines
- anxiety/depression.

Cognitive impairment may affect the patient's ability to understand and communicate with carers and professionals, and to adhere to drug treatment. It places an added burden on those closest to the patient.

SUMMARY

The syndrome of advanced heart failure is the result of complex disturbances of physiology and spares no system of the body. A patient with advanced heart failure will inevitably suffer from most symptoms on the following list:
- fatigue
- breathlessness
- ankle swelling
- disturbed sleep
- difficulty in concentration
- depression
- impaired appetite.

To the extent that these have physical causes, they form the 'doctor's agenda' in heart failure. However, the patient's agenda is considerably broader, as we have already glimpsed in Chapter 1 and will explore in more detail in Chapters 5 ('Symptom relief for advanced heart failure') and 6. Most doctors, while recognising that their main role is in the relief of physical symptoms and the conditions that cause them, will also recognise the need to address the wider needs of the patient. This cannot be done without involving a team of professionals who can interact and communicate effectively.

REFERENCES

1 Baig MK, Mahon N, McKenna WJ et al. The pathophysiology of advanced heart failure. Am Heart J. 1998; **135**(6 Pt 2 Suppl.): S216–30.

2 Najjar SS. Heart failure with preserved ejection fraction: failure to preserve, failure of reserve, and failure on the compliance curve. J Am Coll Cardiol. 2009; **54**(5): 419–21.

3 British Heart Foundation. Prevalence. Available at: www.bhf.org.uk/research/heart-statistics/morbidity/prevalence.aspx (accessed 10 May 2015).

4 Felker GM, O'Connor CM. Inotropic therapy for heart failure: an evidence-based approach. Am Heart J. 2001; **142**(3): 393–401.

5 Velazquez EJ, Lee KL, Deja MA et al. Coronary-artery bypass surgery in patients with left ventricular dysfunction. N Engl J Med. 2011; **364**(17):1607–16.

6 Gaballa MA, Goldman S. Ventricular remodelling in heart failure. J Card Fail. 2002; **8**(6 Suppl.): S476–85.

7 Kostin S, Pool L, Elsässer A et al. Myocytes die by multiple mechanisms in failing human hearts. Circ Res. 2003; **92**(7): 715–24.

8 Maisel WH, Stevenson LW. Atrial fibrillation in heart failure: epidemiology, pathophysiology, and rationale for therapy. Am J Cardiol. 2003; **91**(6A): 2D–8D.

9 McAlister FA, Ezekowitz JA, Wiebe N et al. Systematic review: cardiac resynchronization in patients with symptomatic heart failure. Ann Intern Med. 2004; **141**(5): 381–90.

10 Clark AL. Origin of symptoms in chronic heart failure. Heart. 2006; **92**(1): 12–16.

11 Anker SD, Coats AJ. Cardiac cachexia: a syndrome with impaired survival and immune and neuroendocrine activation. Chest. 1999; **115**(3): 836–47.

12 Sharma R, Anker SD. Cytokines, apoptosis and cachexia: the potential for TNF antagonism. Int J Cardiol. 2002; **85**(1): 161–71.

13 Anker SD, von Haehling S. Inflammatory mediators in chronic heart failure: an overview. Heart. 2004; **90**(4): 464–70.

14 Smart N, Marwick TH. Exercise training for patients with heart failure: a systematic review of factors that improve mortality and morbidity. Am J Med. 2004; **116**(10): 693–706.

15 Leung RS, Bowman ME, Parker JD et al. Avoidance of the left lateral decubitus position during sleep in patients with heart failure: relationship to cardiac size and function. J Am Coll Cardiol. 2003; **41**(2): 227–30

16 Thibodeau JT, Turer AT, Gualano SK et al. Characterization of a novel symptom of advanced heart failure: bendopnea. JACC Heart Fail. 2014; **2**(1):24–31.

17 Ferrier K, Campbell A, Yee B et al. Sleep-disordered breathing occurs frequently in stable outpatients with congestive heart failure. Chest. 2005; **128**(4): 2116–22.

18 Arzt M, Floras JS, Logan AG et al. Suppression of central sleep apnea by continuous positive airway pressure and transplant-free survival in heart failure: a post hoc

analysis of the Canadian Continuous Positive Airway Pressure for Patients with Central Sleep Apnea and Heart Failure Trial (CANPAP). *Circulation.* 2007; **115**(25): 3173-80.

19 Khayat RN, Abraham WT, Patt B *et al.* Cardiac effects of continuous and bilevel positive airway pressure for patients with heart failure and obstructive sleep apnea: a pilot study. *Chest.* 2008; **134**(6): 1162-8.

20 Smith LA, Vennelle M, Gardner RS *et al.* Auto-titrating continuous positive airway pressure therapy in patients with chronic heart failure and obstructive sleep apnoea: a randomized placebo-controlled trial. *Eur Heart J.* 2007; **28**(10): 1221-7.

21 Bradley TD, Logan AG, Kimoff RJ *et al.* Continuous positive airway pressure for central sleep apnea and heart failure. *N Engl J Med.* 2005; **353**(19): 2025-33.

22 Sasayama S, Izumi T, Seino Y *et al.* Effects of nocturnal oxygen therapy on outcome measures in patients with chronic heart failure and Cheyne-Stokes respiration. *Circ J.* 2006; **70**(1): 1-7.

23 Krack A, Sharma R, Figulla HR *et al.* The importance of the gastrointestinal system in the pathogenesis of heart failure. *Eur Heart J.* 2005; **26**(22): 2368-74.

24 Aquilani R, Opasich C, Verri M *et al.* Is nutritional intake adequate in chronic heart failure patients? *J Am Coll Cardiol.* 2003; **42**(7): 1218-23.

25 de Lorgeril M, Salen P, Defaye P. Importance of nutrition in chronic heart failure patients. *Eur Heart J.* 2005; **26**(21): 2215-17.

26 Lindenfeld J. Prevalence of anemia and effects on mortality in patients with heart failure. *Am Heart J.* 2005; **149**(3): 391-401.

27 Pasich C, Cazzola M, Scelsi L *et al.* Blunted erythropoietin production and defective iron supply for erythropoiesis as major causes of anaemia in patients with chronic heart failure. *Eur Heart J.* 2005; **26**(21): 2232-7.

28 van der Meer P, Voors A, Lipsic E *et al.* Erythropoietin in cardiovascular diseases. *Eur Heart J.* 2004; **25**(4): 285-91.

29 Anker SD, Colet JC, Filippatos G *et al.* Ferric carboxymaltose in patients with heart failure and iron deficiency. *N Engl J Med.* 2009; **361**(25): 2436-48.

30 Swedberg K, Young JB, Anand IS *et al.* Treatment of anemia with darbepoetin alfa in systolic heart failure. *N Engl J Med.* 2013; **368**(13): 1210-19.

31 Broström A, Johansson P. Sleep disturbances in patients with chronic heart failure and their holistic consequences: what different care actions can be implemented? *Eur J Cardiovasc Nurs.* 2005; **4**(3): 183-97.

32 MacMahon KM, Lip GY. Psychological factors in heart failure: a review of the literature. *Arch Intern Med.* 2002; **162**(5): 509-16.

33 Konstam V, Moser DK, De Jong MJ. Depression and anxiety in heart failure. *J Card Fail.* 2005; **11**(6): 455-63.

34 Gottlieb SS, Khatta M, Friedmann E *et al.* The influence of age, gender, and race on the prevalence of depression in heart failure patients. *J Am Coll Cardiol.* 2004; **43**(9): 1542-9.

35 Pasic J, Levy WC, Sullivan MD. Cytokines in depression and heart failure. *Psychosom Med.* 2003; **65**(2): 181-93.

36 Fekertich AK, Ferguson JP, Binkley PF. Depressive symptoms and inflammation among heart failure patients. *Am Heart J.* 2005; **150**(1): 132-6.

37 Genth-Zotz S, von Haehling S, Bolger AP *et al.* Pathophysiologic quantities of

endotoxin-induced tumor necrosis factor-alpha release in whole blood from patients with chronic heart failure. *Am J Cardiol.* 2002; **90**(11): 1226–30.

38 Woo MJ, Macey PM, Keens PT *et al.* Functional abnormalities in brain areas that mediate autonomic nervous system control in advanced heart failure. *J Card Fail.* 2005; **11**(6): 437–46.

CHAPTER 3

Optimal therapy for heart failure

SHONA JENKINS

INTRODUCTION

The medical management of heart failure with reduced ejection fraction is supported by a substantial evidence base, with clear morbidity and mortality benefits demonstrated for drugs, in various classes, targeting the deleterious effects of 'compensatory' neurohumoral activation to reduced cardiac function. Notably, the clinical trial populations have been predominantly male with a mean age of 60–65 years. Consequently, the evidence for medical therapy in heart failure in older people with multiple co-morbidities is less robust. However, this distinction is not reflected in national or international guidance for heart failure management. The cornerstones of heart failure medical therapy are angiotensin-converting enzyme (ACE) inhibitors (or angiotensin receptor blockers), beta-adrenoceptor antagonists, mineralocorticoid receptor antagonists (MRAs) and diuretics. A number of other pharmacological and non-pharmacological therapies may be appropriate for selected patients, including implantable cardiovertor defibrillators (ICDs) and cardiac resynchronisation therapy (CRT) pacemakers.

Importantly, it should be recognised that the evidence base for both pharmacological and non-pharmacological therapy in heart failure is specific to patients with heart failure and reduced ejection fraction, with no studies to date demonstrating significant morbidity or mortality benefit in heart failure with preserved ejection fraction, despite similar clinical presentation, symptom burden and prognosis. As such, the mainstay of medical management in these patients is diuretics to minimise recurrent pulmonary congestion and peripheral oedema. Notably, heart failure with preserved ejection fraction is more common in older people.

The disease trajectory in chronic heart failure is unpredictable, and, as such, prognostication is extremely difficult. However, there are various indicators of very poor prognosis, such as persistent New York Heart Association (NYHA) class IV symptoms despite optimal heart failure therapy, recurrent hospital admission with cardiac decompensation and the development of cardiac cachexia. As heart failure becomes more advanced and end of life approaches, the focus of evidence-based pharmacological and non-pharmacological therapy shifts from reducing mortality to effectively managing symptoms, minimising psychological distress, anticipatory care planning and meeting patients' priorities and preferences of care.

This chapter describes the standard medical management of heart failure with reduced ejection fraction and offers a practical guide to the initiation and titration of therapy. Specific consideration is given to specific patient cohorts for which the evidence base is lacking and a more pragmatic approach is required; for example, older patients with multiple co-morbidities. There is subsequent discussion of appropriate optimisation of pharmacological therapy in advanced heart failure and as end of life approaches. The indications for device therapy (ICDs and CRT), mechanical circulatory support and transplantation are presented with discussion thereafter of the issues surrounding elective device deactivation in end-stage heart failure.

STANDARD MEDICAL THERAPY
Diuretics

Diuretics are essential in the management of heart failure to ameliorate symptomatic pulmonary and peripheral congestion. Loop diuretics (frusemide, bumetanide, torasemide) and thiazide or thiazide-like diuretics (bendroflumethiazide, metolazone) exert their effect on the loop of Henle and the distal tubule, respectively, to promote sodium and water loss. Intravenous frusemide is standard therapy in the management of decompensated heart failure. Most patients require maintenance therapy with an oral loop diuretic and, for many, a supplemental thiazide or thiazide-like diuretic is needed. While only a handful of small placebo-controlled studies has assessed the clinical benefits of diuretics in chronic heart failure, the available evidence is suggestive of both morbidity and mortality benefit.[1]

Initiation of diuretic therapy in a stable patient with heart failure is usually with oral frusemide at a dose of 40 mg. This can then be titrated as required to achieve and maintain euvolaemia while avoiding excessive volume depletion and pre-renal impairment. Common titrated doses of frusemide are 80 mg or 120 mg twice daily. Higher doses may be required in patients with significant renal impairment. Bumetanide is often used when higher doses of frusemide are ineffective. It is better absorbed from the intestine, particularly in the context of gut oedema. Bumetanide 1 mg is equivalent to 40 mg of frusemide for a patient with normal renal function. Common titrated doses are 2 mg or 3 mg twice daily. Concomitant synergistic thiazide therapy with bendroflumethiazide 2.5–5.0 mg or metolazone 2.5–5.0 mg, either daily, on alternate days or once or twice weekly may be required in patients with resistant oedema despite loop-diuretic titration. In practical terms, the addition of a thiazide is often beneficial with respect to managing resistant fluid overload once frusemide 80 mg twice daily (bumetanide 2 mg twice daily) is ineffective.

Once stable, patients are encouraged to maintain euvolaemia by adhering to a fluid restriction (usually 1.5 L to 2.0 L daily) and by monitoring their weight with small adjustments in their diuretic dose as required. A useful indicator is an increase of 2 kg in weight over a 3-day period or the detection by the patient of a recurrence of peripheral oedema. In these instances, it may be considered reasonable for the patient to manage their own diuretic dose and so, for example, to increase the dose of frusemide by an additional 40 mg daily until their optimal weight is regained. This may be done autonomously or in collaboration with a specialist heart failure nurse.

Recognition of over-diuresis is important, and the tired patient with dizziness on standing and a corresponding postural drop in blood pressure should have their loop-diuretic dose reviewed. It should be remembered that hyponatraemia may be representative of over-diuresis or of haemodilution due to decompensated heart failure with fluid overload, and so must be interpreted in the clinical context. Diuretic dosage may need to be reduced in hot climates if patients travel abroad or, similarly, decreased in the context of intercurrent illness with diarrhoea or vomiting. Avoidance of hypokalaemia is important; although, in a euvolaemic patient, this can often be managed by titration of renin–angiotensin–aldosterone system (RAAS) blocking drugs, which is eminently desirable in the management of heart failure.

Summary points: diuretics

- Most patients require maintenance therapy with a loop diuretic, and many can be managed well on frusemide alone.
- Bumetanide is a useful alternative to frusemide in resistant oedema when there is concern about intestinal absorption.
- Synergistic thiazide therapy with bendroflumethiazide or metolazone may help promote diuresis and maintain euvolaemia.
- Careful monitoring of renal function and electrolytes is important.
- Loop diuretics can be self-managed by patients who have been taught to monitor their weight.
- Over-diuresis can precipitate postural dizziness and fatigue.

ACE INHIBITORS AND ANGIOTENSIN RECEPTOR BLOCKERS
ACE inhibitors

Multiple large, randomised, double-blind, placebo-controlled clinical trials have irrefutably demonstrated the beneficial effects of ACE inhibitors (enalapril, captopril, lisinopril, ramipril, trandolapril) in heart failure with reduced ejection fraction.[2-7] There is unequivocal evidence of mortality benefit and morbidity benefit in terms of improving NYHA class and reducing hospital admissions. ACE inhibitors inhibit the RAAS by reducing the production of angiotensin II and slowing the breakdown of bradykinin. This results in vasodilatation, with a consequent reduction in afterload and myocardial work. The downstream production of aldosterone is diminished, which promotes sodium and water loss. RAAS inhibition is also considered to ameliorate adverse ventricular remodelling. As such, ACE inhibitors are first-line medical therapy in all patients with heart failure, irrespective of NYHA class.

What is the optimum dose?

ACE inhibitors should be initiated at a low dose with subsequent up-titration over weeks or months to the maximum-tolerated dose, up to the top doses achieved in clinical trials. While some ACE inhibitor is inherently better than no ACE inhibitor, there is evidence that higher doses confer greater benefit – at least with respect to reduction in heart failure-related hospital admissions and reports of worsening heart failure, although with no associated significant difference in survival or change in symptomatic functional status.[6] Titration may be impeded by symptomatic hypotension or by deteriorating renal function, and, indeed, the Assessment of Treatment with Lisinopril and Survival (ATLAS) study trial confirmed that those allocated to high dose (32.5–35.0 mg lisinopril) had more hypotension, dizziness, worsening renal function and hyperkalaemia than those taking low dose (2.5–5.0 mg). However, the investigators reported that these effects were managed straightforwardly with either dose adjustments of the lisinopril or rationalisation of other medication.[6] The lack of effect on survival between high- and low-dose regimens is consistently seen,[8] thus the approach must be one of aiming for the optimally tolerated dose to minimise hospital admissions with decompensation, rather than a 'target-dose-at-all-costs' strategy with a promise of increased survival.

First-dose hypotension can be predicted in the context of a resting tachycardia, existing hypotension, hyponatraemia, concomitant vasodilator therapy (e.g. oral nitrates) and unstable heart failure. Therefore, achieving euvolaemia prior to ACE-inhibitor initiation is important. Nocturnal dosing is a useful strategy when initiation or titration is limited by hypotension. Careful monitoring for renal impairment and hyperkalaemia is important during ACE-inhibitor titration. Some deterioration in renal function is common, and international guidance considers a rise in creatinine up to 50% above baseline (provided the creatinine level remains <266 μmol) to be acceptable.[9] In practice, a reduction in loop-diuretic dose often permits further escalation of ACE-inhibitor therapy while preserving renal function without precipitating decompensation.

Contraindications to ACE-inhibitor initiation are: existing hyperkalaemia, bilateral renal artery stenosis, severe aortic stenosis, severe renal impairment without renal replacement therapy (estimated Glomerular filtration rate (GFR) <30 mL/min/1.73 m²), pregnancy and previous intolerance due to angio-oedema or ACE inhibitor-induced cough. An ACE inhibitor-induced cough, occurring in 5%–10% patients, is the result of impaired bradykinin clearance from the upper airway and is a class effect of all the ACE inhibitors.

What about older people?

Given the importance of a greater focus on quality of life rather than survival in older people, it is notable that less than 30% of the patients in the clinical trials of ACE inhibitors were over the age of 70, and so the effects of standard medical therapy on those over 75 years are not easy to ascertain.[10] A pooled individual analysis of data from ACE-inhibitor trials relating to a subgroup of those over 75 years old did not find evidence of benefit for clinical outcomes, but this was considered to be a feature of low numbers.[11]

Angiotensin receptor blockers

Angiotensin receptor blockers (ARBs) inhibit the RAAS by specifically antagonising the angiotensin II receptor, type 1 (or 'AT1 receptor'). This action promotes vasodilatation and sodium and water excretion while reducing antidiuretic hormone release. Since ARBs do not inhibit bradykinin breakdown, the adverse effects associated with ACE inhibitors, such as cough and angio-oedema, are far less common. Thus, an ARB is considered an appropriate alternative for a patient intolerant of ACE inhibition.

There is a substantial body of evidence confirming the mortality and morbidity benefits of ARBs (valsartan, candesartan, losartan) in heart failure with reduced ejection fraction.[12–15] Two studies have demonstrated additional morbidity benefit when an ARB is added to baseline ACE-inhibitor therapy.[15,16] International guidance recommended this approach for a period, but with the emerging evidence supporting MRA therapy in combination with ACE inhibition to reduce mortality in heart failure, dual therapy with an ACE inhibitor and an ARB is only considered potentially appropriate if there is MRA intolerance.[9] Triple RAAS blockade with an ACE inhibitor, an MRA and an ARB is not recommended due to the inherent risk of renal dysfunction and significant hyperkalaemia.

The process of initiation and titration of an ARB is no different to that of an ACE inhibitor. The starting dose should be small, with incremental up-titration, as tolerated by blood pressure and renal function, over several weeks, aiming for the maximum-tolerated dose up to a maximum of those achieved in the clinical trials.

What about older people?

Those over the age of 65 years appear to be just as likely to receive benefit from ARBs as their younger counterparts,[17] but there is still no significant evidence of beneficial effects in those over 80 years old.

Hydralazine and nitrates

Combination therapy with hydralazine and isosorbide dinitrate (H-ISDN) is often prescribed for patients intolerant of both ACE inhibitors and ARBs. Hydralazine is an arteriolar dilator, exerting a positive effect on cardiac output by reducing afterload. Isosorbide dinitrate is a venodilator at lower doses, reducing preload, but has arteriolar dilating properties at higher doses. Large RCTs demonstrated that H-ISDN reduces all-cause mortality in heart failure in comparison to placebo but to a lesser extent than ACE inhibition.[18,19] A further study confirmed additional morbidity and mortality benefit for H-ISDN in

African Americans already established on ACE inhibitors.[20] Therefore, international guidance recommends H-ISDN for patients who are intolerant of ACE inhibitors and ARBs and for African American patients who remain symptomatic despite an ACE inhibitor or ARB.[9]

Initiation of H-ISDN is usually with hydralazine 25 mg four times daily along with isosorbide dinitrate 10 mg four times daily. Titration is to a maximum dose of hydralazine 75 mg four times daily and isosorbide dinitrate 40 mg four times daily, but this is rarely achieved in clinical practice, with dose escalation often limited by symptomatic hypotension and headache.

Summary points: ACE inhibitors, ARBs and H-ISDN

- Large RCTs have unequivocally demonstrated that, in comparison to placebo, ACE inhibitors and ARBs reduce morbidity and mortality in patients with heart failure and reduced ejection fraction, irrespective of NYHA class.
- Initiation of an ACE inhibitor or ARB should be at a low dose, with up-titration as tolerated by blood pressure and renal function up to the maximum doses achieved in the clinical trials.

Higher doses of ACE inhibitors are associated with a reduction in heart failure-related admissions but not with increased survival.

- 'First-dose hypotension' is more common in the context of resting tachycardia, existing hypotension, hyponatraemia, concomitant vasodilator therapy (e.g. oral nitrates) and unstable heart failure.
- Titration of an ACE inhibitor or ARB may facilitate a reduction in loop-diuretic dose.
- Five to ten per cent of patients do not tolerate an ACE inhibitor due to a dry cough so should instead be commenced on an ARB.
- An ACE inhibitor should only be given in combination with an ARB in symptomatic patients who are intolerant of an MRA.
- H-ISDN is an alternative evidenced-based therapy for patients who are intolerant of ACE inhibitors and ARBs.

BETA-ADRENOCEPTOR ANTAGONISTS (BETA-BLOCKERS)

Multiple large RCTs have unequivocally demonstrated the substantial morbidity and mortality benefits conferred by beta-blocker therapy in heart failure with reduced ejection fraction.[21-5] By counteracting the deleterious effects of the sympathetic nervous system, they have been shown to improve cardiac function and NYHA class, while reducing all-cause mortality, including sudden cardiac death. International guidance recommends commencement of a beta-blocker (in addition to an ACE inhibitor or ARB) in all patients with heart failure, irrespective of NYHA class.[9] The specific beta-blockers with a clear evidence base in heart failure are carvedilol, bisoprolol and metoprolol sustained release. Similarly to ACE inhibitors, a low dose is initiated followed by cautious titration as tolerated over weeks or months, up to the maximum doses used in the clinical trials. Careful monitoring of heart rate, blood pressure and fluid status is essential, and the risk of cardiac decompensation following introduction or dose escalation of a beta-blocker is well recognised. Therefore, it is essential that euvolaemia and clinical stability be achieved before initiation of a beta-blocker. Importantly, a resting sinus tachycardia is an indicator of unstable heart failure, even if seemingly euvolaemic, and initiation of a beta-blocker in that context should be avoided. In stable chronic heart failure, beta-blockers are also useful in the ventricular rate control of atrial fibrillation (AF). Interestingly, however, a recent individual patient data meta-analysis of 10 RCTs demonstrated that the morbidity and mortality benefits of beta-blockers seen in patients with heart failure and reduced ejection fraction in sinus rhythm are not seen in those with AF, irrespective of age, gender, left ventricular ejection fraction, NYHA class or baseline medical therapy.[26]

Contraindications to commencing a beta-blocker are second- or third-degree heart block, critical peripheral vascular disease and asthma. Chronic obstructive pulmonary disease (COPD) is not considered a contraindication to cardio-selective beta-blockade.[9] However, caution would seem appropriate in severe COPD with significant reversibility. While a beta-blocker should never be initiated in the context of decompensated heart failure, decompensation should not prompt discontinuation of a beta-blocker that has previously been tolerated. Indeed, due to up-regulation of beta-adrenoceptors during beta-blocker treatment, abrupt discontinuation may precipitate arrhythmia, angina or a further reduction in cardiac function. A dose reduction is often appropriate, particularly if there is hypotension, and escalation of diuretic therapy is essential, with intravenous diuretic sometimes required.

What about older people?

Older patients are less able to tolerate beta-blockers. As with ACE-inhibitor trials, less than 30% of trial participants have been over the age of 70 years, with very few over the age of 80 years. However, subgroup analyses have demonstrated a relationship between age and beta-blocker study outcomes.[27] An RCT of the beta-blocker nebivolol in patients over 70 years showed benefit in the primary combined endpoint of mortality and hospitalisation, but less so than other beta-blocker trials that included younger patients, and did not show a benefit for mortality alone.[28] Subgroup analysis of those over 75 years did not show benefit in primary outcome.

Summary points: beta-adrenoceptor antagonists (beta-blockers)

- Multiple large RCTs have irrefutably demonstrated the substantial morbidity and mortality benefits conferred by beta-blocker therapy in heart failure in patients under the age of 75 years.
- Beta-blockade should be initiated after the patient is euvolaemic on oral diuretic and established on an ACE inhibitor.
- Beta-blocker dose escalation should be slow, with vigilance for symptoms and signs suggestive of cardiac decompensation, which may require up-titration of diuretics.

- In the context of cardiac decompensation in a patient already established on a beta-blocker, discontinuation should be avoided, but a dose reduction may be appropriate.
- Beta-blockers are contraindicated in patients with asthma but are not contraindicated in COPD.

Beta-blockers are unlikely to confer mortality benefit in patients with heart failure and concomitant AF but are still useful in ventricular rate control.

MRAs

ACE inhibitors (or ARBs) do not reliably suppress aldosterone production. Indeed, it is well recognised that 'aldosterone escape' occurs in up to 40% of patients with chronic heart failure. Excess aldosterone in heart failure is associated with adverse cardiac remodelling, ventricular arrhythmia and increased mortality. Spironolactone and eplerenone are MRAs that competitively inhibit the effects of aldosterone. There is now clear evidence from large RCTs to support the addition of an MRA to standard therapy with an ACE inhibitor (or ARB) and a beta-blocker to confer further morbidity and mortality benefit in patients with NYHA class II–IV heart failure.[29,30] Additionally, eplerenone has been proven to improve outcomes in a post-myocardial infarction (MI) population with left ventricular systolic dysfunction and either clinical heart failure or diabetes.[31] Spironolactone is a non-selective aldosterone antagonist that binds to androgen and progesterone receptors, so is associated with gynaecomastia and menstrual irregularities in men and women, respectively. Eplerenone is a newer selective mineralocorticoid antagonist that causes less gynaecomastia.

In practice, an MRA should be introduced when symptoms persist despite maximum-tolerated therapy with an ACE inhibitor and a beta-blocker. Both spironolactone and eplerenone are usually commenced at a dose of 25 mg with up-titration to 50 mg if tolerated with respect to blood pressure, renal dysfunction and, in particular, hyperkalaemia. A starting dose of 12.5 mg can be used if there is concern about symptomatic hypotension. Careful monitoring of renal function and for hyperkalaemia (abnormally high potassium levels) is essential, and it is prudent to check potassium levels at 1 week and 3 weeks following each dose change.

What about older people?

Subgroup analysis of the Randomised ALdactone Evaluation (RALES) study did not show a difference in outcome between those above and below the age of 67 years.[29] However, it is well documented that adverse effects are more common in older people.[32]

Summary points: MRAs

- Evidence from RCTs supports the addition of an MRA to established therapy

with an ACE inhibitor (or ARB) and a beta-blocker to further reduce morbidity and mortality in patients with NYHA class II–IV heart failure.
- Spironolactone is a non-selective aldosterone antagonist that may cause gynaecomastia in men.
- Eplerenone is a selective aldosterone antagonist that is much less likely to cause gynaecomastia.
- Renal function and, in particular, potassium levels must be carefully monitored during MRA initiation and titration.

DIGOXIN AND IVABRADINE
Digoxin

Digoxin, a cardiac glycoside, has a weak inotropic effect and properties that slow conduction across the atrioventricular node. The Digitalis Investigation Group (DIG) trial demonstrated that the addition of digoxin in patients with chronic heart failure established on ACE inhibitors conferred additional clinical benefit by reducing the risk of hospitalisation due to decompensated heart failure.[33] However, there was no additional mortality benefit. A post-hoc analysis demonstrated the optimum digoxin concentration to be 0.5–0.8 ng/mL to maximise morbidity benefit while minimising complications such as digitoxicity.[34] International guidance recommends the addition of digoxin if patients remain symptomatic despite maximal-tolerated ACE inhibitor (or ARB), beta-blocker and MRA.[9] Digoxin also has a role to play in ventricular rate control in AF when a beta-blocker is either insufficient to control rate or is otherwise contraindicated. Of note, AF is common in chronic heart failure, affecting up to 27% of patients with significant heart failure.[35] A recent retrospective cohort study examining the use of digoxin in patients older than 65 years with AF both with and without heart failure found an increase in all-cause mortality in both groups.[36] However, this has not yet been demonstrated in either a prospective cohort study or an RCT.

It is important to avoid hypokalaemia in the context of digoxin therapy, as this increases the risk of toxicity and arrhythmia. Women, older people and those with renal impairment are particularly at risk. It should also be remembered that digoxin concentrations can be increased due to interactions with other common drugs taken by patients with chronic heart failure (e.g. spironolactone and amiodarone). For patients who are anticoagulated with warfarin, the addition of digoxin often necessitates an increase in warfarin dose to maintain a therapeutic international normalised ratio. Digoxin should be initiated at a daily dose dependent on renal function (usually between 62.5 μg and 250.0 μg daily). 'Loading doses' of digoxin are not required unless the goal is to rapidly control ventricular rate in AF. Careful monitoring of digoxin levels is required due to the narrow therapeutic window that avoids toxicity and due to the precarious renal function that often exists in patients with chronic heart failure. Digoxin has multiple well-recognised side effects, including nausea, dizziness and visual disturbance, which often limit use.

What about older people?

Data from the DIG study did not show any significant relationships between age and digoxin treatment with respect to any of the major clinical end points, but older patients were more likely to experience adverse events, in particular, increased hospital admissions with suspected toxicity.[37]

Ivabradine

Ivabradine is a direct sino-atrial node inhibitor that lowers heart rate without affecting blood pressure. The Systolic Heart failure treatment with the I_f inhibitor ivabradine Trial (SHIFT) study compared ivabradine with placebo in patients with chronic heart failure already established on maximal-tolerated evidence-based therapy with ACE inhibitors (or ARBs), beta-blockers and MRAs.[38] It demonstrated a significant reduction in relative risk of a composite end point of cardiovascular death or hospital admission with decompensated heart failure (driven by the latter). The study received criticism because only just over half the participants were on 50% or more of target beta-blocker dose. As such, it is not clear whether the benefit of ivabradine would have persisted had beta-blockers been titrated to maximum dose. While hypotension may limit the titration of beta-blockers, the mean systolic blood pressure at entry to SHIFT was 122 mmHg, suggesting further escalation of beta-blockade may have been possible. Ivabradine is approved for use in patients with heart failure in several countries across Europe including the UK and recently the US Food and Drug Administration approved its use in the USA. The European Society of Cardiology (ESC) supports ivabradine in symptomatic patients with an ejection fraction of less than 35% and a heart rate of 70 bpm or more who cannot tolerate further escalation of beta-blocker therapy, who have already achieved maximum dose or for who a beta-blocker is otherwise contraindicated.[9] However, more recently, the safety of ivabradine has been called into question due to an apparent increased risk of developing AF and a higher risk of cardiovascular events in patients with heart rates less than 70 bpm.[39]

Since the mechanism of action of ivabradine is an effect on the sino-atrial node, it cannot be utilised in the context of AF. The starting dose is 5.0 mg twice daily or 2.5 mg twice daily in older patients or those with significant renal dysfunction. Titration can be up to 7.5 mg twice daily if needed and tolerated. Significant side effects are uncommon but include headache, dizziness and visual disturbance.

Summary points: digoxin and ivabradine

- International guidance supports the addition of digoxin to patients with chronic heart failure who remain symptomatic despite maximal-tolerated therapy with an ACE inhibitor (or ARB), beta-blocker or MRA.
- Digoxin is useful in the control of ventricular rate in AF when a beta-blocker is either not sufficient or not tolerated.
- It is important that digoxin and potassium levels, along with renal function, are monitored to minimise the risk of toxicity.

- Digoxin interacts with some cardiac drugs including amiodarone and spironolactone (increased digoxin concentration) and warfarin (reduced international normalised ratio).
- Side effects of digoxin include nausea, dizziness and visual disturbance.
- To reduce the risk of hospitalisation with decompensation, ivabradine is recommended in Europe (but not the USA) for patients with chronic heart failure in sinus rhythm who are symptomatic despite maximum-tolerated ACE inhibitor (or ARB), beta-blocker and MRA with a resting heart rate of 70 bpm or more.

ASPIRIN AND WARFARIN

The most common cause of heart failure is coronary artery disease, but while aspirin therapy has a robust evidence base for patients with angina and following MI, its use in the context of heart failure is somewhat controversial. First, there has been concern that aspirin might interfere with the actions of ACE inhibitors by blocking prostaglandin synthesis.[4] However, in the most recent (and largest) study of anti-platelet and anticoagulant therapy in heart failure, warfarin versus aspirin in reduced cardiac ejection fraction (WARCEF) study, there was no evidence to suggest any clinically significant interaction between aspirin and ACE inhibitors.[40] The anti-platelet drug clopidogrel does not affect prostaglandin synthesis, and a study comparing it with aspirin therapy in patients with chronic heart failure is ongoing. At present, international guidance supports continuation of anti-platelet therapy in heart failure when coronary artery disease coexists, but it is not recommended in patients with heart failure of a non-ischaemic aetiology.[9]

In the absence of a significant contraindication, patients with heart failure and coexistent AF (paroxysmal, persistent or permanent) should be anticoagulated with warfarin to reduce the risk of stroke. Warfarin is also considered appropriate in patients with chronic heart failure and sinus rhythm in the context of left ventricular thrombus or if there is a large area of akinetic myocardium with stagnant blood flow.[9] Intuitively, it might seem that anticoagulation would reduce embolic stroke risk in all patients with chronic heart failure and sinus rhythm, since, mechanistically, all three components of Virchow's triad are met (slow blood flow, impaired endothelial activity and a hypercoagulable state). However, the recent WARCEF study demonstrated that, while warfarin was superior to aspirin with respect to reducing ischaemic stroke in patients with chronic heart failure and sinus rhythm, any true clinical benefit was offset by the significantly higher rate of major bleeding complications in the warfarin group.[40] As such, warfarin is not recommended for patients with chronic heart failure in sinus rhythm without an existing recognised indication for anticoagulation.

SUMMARY OF STANDARD MEDICAL THERAPY

The ESC (2012) has produced clear guidance for pharmacological therapy in chronic heart failure.[9] All patients with chronic heart failure with reduced ejection fraction, irrespective of NYHA class, should be established on an ACE inhibitor (or ARB if there is ACE-inhibitor intolerance due to cough) and a beta-blocker with an evidence base in heart failure. The doses should be titrated as tolerated by renal function, heart rate and blood pressure, up to the top doses achieved in clinical trials. Combination therapy with H-ISDN is an alternative strategy for those intolerant of both ACE inhibitors and ARBs. To maintain euvolaemia, most patients will require an oral loop diuretic, and some may need occasional or regular thiazide diuretic therapy. If symptoms persist despite euvolaemia and maximum-tolerated ACE inhibitor (or ARB) and beta-blocker, the addition of an MRA is appropriate, with careful monitoring of renal function and potassium levels. The morbidity and mortality benefits conferred by ACE inhibitors (or ARBs), beta-blockers and MRAs are additive. When dose titration of these drugs is limited by symptomatic hypotension, the aim should be to establish patients on a small dose of each rather than a large dose of one drug and none of the others. Patients who remain symptomatic despite triple therapy with an ACE inhibitor (or an ARB), a beta-blocker and an MRA can be commenced on digoxin, which also has a more specific role in ventricular rate control in AF when beta-blockade alone is either insufficient or not tolerated. Ivabradine may be considered in patients in sinus rhythm when a beta-blocker is contraindicated or when titration is impeded by symptomatic hypotension. Aspirin is appropriate for patients with chronic heart failure and coexistent coronary artery disease, and warfarin should be given to reduce stroke risk in AF unless otherwise contraindicated. Warfarin should only be given (unless otherwise indicated, e.g. mechanical heart valves) to patients with chronic heart failure in sinus rhythm if there is evidence of left ventricular thrombus.

DECOMPENSATED HEART FAILURE

Even in the context of optimal evidence-based medical therapy as outlined earlier, recurrent decompensation of heart failure is common, and decompensation requiring hospital admission is well recognised to be a poor prognostic sign. Mild decompensation with worsening peripheral or pulmonary congestion can often be managed in primary care by up-titration of oral diuretics, perhaps facilitated by a specialist heart failure nurse. More significant decompensation and acute cardiac decompensation usually necessitates admission to hospital. Medical therapy then variably includes supplemental oxygen (including non-invasive continuous positive airway pressure ventilation), intravenous opioids, diuretic and nitrates with or without inotropic support, usually in the form of intravenous dopamine and dobutamine. Ceilings of therapy should be considered and, in specific selected cases, intra-aortic balloon counter pulsation may be appropriate, usually in a context in which mechanical circulatory support and/or cardiac transplantation would be a plausible exit strategy (*see* the following section, 'Device therapy').

Determining the cause of an episode of cardiac decompensation is important. Common causes include intercurrent infection, transient or sustained arrhythmia (AF, ventricular tachycardia), acute coronary syndrome, pulmonary thromboembolism, non-compliance with heart failure medication, new inappropriate medication (e.g. non-steroidal anti-inflammatory drugs or non-dihydropyridine calcium-channel antagonists), anaemia, hyperthyroidism or uncontrolled diabetes. After rendering the decompensated patient euvolaemic and considering and treating any precipitating cause, it is usually appropriate to up-titrate heart failure medical therapy, if tolerated, to minimise the risk of further decompensation. Recurrent cardiac decompensation requiring hospital admission suggests a very poor prognosis, so should prompt discussions regarding ceilings of treatment and the patient's priorities and preferences of care.

DEVICE THERAPY
CRT

Cardiac resynchronisation therapy pacing (CRT-P) aims to reduce the interventricular dyssynchrony and atrioventricular conduction delay that occur in heart failure. The cardiac resynchronisation-heart failure (CARE-HF) trial was the landmark clinical trial in 2005 that clearly demonstrated a mortality benefit for CRT-P in patients with NYHA class III–IV chronic heart failure, a left ventricular ejection fraction of less than 35% and a left bundle-branch block (LBBB) pattern with QRS duration equal to or greater than 150 ms (or >120 ms with echocardiographic evidence of mechanical dyssynchrony).[41] Significant improvements in NYHA class and in quality-of-life scores were also demonstrated in the CRT-P group. Subsequent studies have determined that CRT-P confers morbidity and mortality benefits in patients with NYHA class II heart failure and ejection fraction less than 30% and in patients with NYHA class I–II heart failure and ejection fraction less than 50% with a pacing indication that would precipitate persistent right ventricular pacing.[42-4] It appears that LBBB and a QRS duration of longer than 150 ms are associated with the best response to CRT-P. There is limited evidence for CRT-P in the context of a QRS duration of less than 130 ms, right bundle-branch block morphology and in AF. The use of echocardiography to assess mechanical dyssynchrony with a view to improving patient selection for CRT-P is no longer considered useful.[45] The ESC recommendations for CRT-P therapy in chronic heart failure vary depending on whether there is NYHA class II or III–IV heart failure, LBBB or non-LBBB morphology, and sinus rhythm or AF. A CRT defibrillator (i.e. cardiac resynchronisation therapy defibrillation [CRT-D]), as opposed to a CRT pacemaker, is implanted if the patient also meets the criteria for defibrillator therapy (*see* the following section, 'ICDs'). Table 3.1 summarises the most recent ESC guidance (2012) for CRT-P/D implantation when there is considered to be a strong

TABLE 3.1 Indications for cardiac resynchronisation therapy pacing/defibrillation (CRT-P/D) with a strong evidence base

	NYHA class II		NYHA class III–IV	
	LBBB	**Non-LBBB**	**LBBB**	**Non-LBBB**
QRS (ms)	≥130	≥150	≥120	>150
Rhythm	Sinus	Sinus	Sinus	Sinus
EF (%)	≤30	≤30	≤35	≤35
CRT-P/CRT-D	Ideally CRT-D	Ideally CRT-D	CRT-P/CRT-D	CRT-P/CRT-D

EF = ejection fraction; LBBB = left bundle-branch block; NYHA = New York Heart Association.
Source: Adapted from McMurray *et al.*[9]

evidence base.[9] The ESC also supports CRT-P implantation in AF with an ejection fraction of 35% or less, a QRS duration of 120 ms or longer and NYHA class III–IV heart failure if the heart rate is sufficiently slow (<60 bpm at rest and <90 bpm with exercise) or if pacing is required. CRT-P should also be considered in the context of NYHA class II–IV heart failure with ejection fraction of 35% or lower, irrespective of QRS duration, if there is a permanent pacing indication.

ICDs

Sudden cardiac death occurs in around half of patients with heart failure and the majority of this can be attributed to ventricular arrhythmia, which is common despite optimal heart failure therapy with neurohumoral antagonists. ICDs have been demonstrated to improve survival in both primary and secondary prevention in patients with both ischaemic and non-ischaemic chronic heart failure.[46-8] Sudden cardiac death in heart failure trial (SCD-HeFT), a primary prevention trial in NYHA class II–III chronic heart failure, demonstrated that an ICD reduced the relative risk of death by 22% in comparison to placebo, while the class III anti-arrhythmic amiodarone was no better than placebo and conferred harm in the NYHA class III subgroup.[48] The ESC considers the implantation of an ICD appropriate for secondary prevention in survivors of ventricular fibrillation or patients with haemodynamically unstable ventricular tachycardia and survival expectation of more than 1 year. The criteria for primary prevention are NYHA class II–III chronic heart failure with a left ventricular ejection fraction of 35% or less with survival expectation greater than 1 year. In the context of an ischaemic aetiology of heart failure, the patient must be at least 40 days post-MI.[9]

Mechanical circulatory support and cardiac transplantation

While a detailed consideration of mechanical circulatory support (ventricular assist devices, artificial hearts) and cardiac transplantation is outside the scope of this book, it is important to recognise that these options exist for selected patients in specific circumstances. Presently, the most common indication for a ventricular assist device is in acutely decompensated severe heart failure refractory to conventional optimal therapy as a bridge to cardiac transplantation. Short-term mechanical circulatory support should also be considered as a bridge to recovery in severely hypoperfused patients despite inotropic therapy when there is a potential reversible or surgically correctable cause (e.g. viral myocarditis or acute inter-ventricular septal rupture). While there is some evidence to support mechanical circulatory support as destination therapy in specific patients ineligible for transplantation, experience of this is limited.[49,50] Cardiac transplantation is a realistic option for a small percentage of carefully selected patients with advanced heart failure refractory to optimal therapy. However, it does have its own significant associated morbidity and mortality.

OPTIMAL MEDICAL THERAPY IN ADVANCED DISEASE APPROACHING END OF LIFE

It is well recognised that the prognosis in heart failure is extremely poor, with over 50% of patients diagnosed with heart failure dying within 5 years. However, the disease trajectory is extremely unpredictable, and, consequently, accurate prognostication is notoriously difficult. While the general trajectory is downward, patients often oscillate between periods of stability (despite limiting symptoms) and recurrent episodes of severe life-threatening decompensation. Sudden cardiac death can occur at any point. Despite the inherent difficulties with accurate prognostication, there are various recognised indicators of advanced disease with a very poor prognosis. These include persistent NYHA class IV symptoms despite optimal therapy, recurrent hospital admissions with cardiac decompensation and the development of cardiac cachexia. In such advanced disease, the focus of therapy shifts somewhat from reducing mortality to effectively managing symptoms and minimising psychological distress, alongside addressing issues surrounding anticipatory care planning and meeting patients' priorities and preferences of care. While a holistic model of care with effective palliation of both physical and psychosocial distress is important throughout the course of heart failure, the role of palliative care undoubtedly becomes increasingly relevant with progression to advanced disease and as end of life approaches.

In general terms, conventional heart failure pharmacological therapy should be continued despite progressive advanced heart failure, provided the morbidity benefits continue to outweigh the drug-related adverse effects. While the mortality benefits of evidence-based therapy lose relevance in very advanced disease, it must be remembered that these drugs have also been shown to alleviate symptoms, enhance well-being and minimise hospital admissions, all of which remain important in advanced disease and when approaching end of life. However, often modifications to pharmacological therapy are required as patients with very advanced disease are more prone to hypovolaemia, hypotension and deteriorating renal function. These factors may necessitate down-titration of various drugs and the continuing regimen needs to be tailored to each individual patient's clinical condition and requirements. For example, diuretics would be continued at the expense of an ACE inhibitor in a patient with painful peripheral oedema, particularly in the context of worsening renal dysfunction; beta-blockers might be prioritised in patients prone to angina. Continuing a beta-blocker may also be important in the context of recurrent ventricular arrhythmia to avoid cardiac decompensation or discharges from an active ICD (*see* the following section, 'Device therapy in advanced disease and approaching end of life'). The addition of oral or transdermal nitrates may be useful in the context of worsening angina. Other therapies to alleviate persistent symptoms become increasingly important, such as opioids, anxiolytics and home oxygen. These are discussed in detail in Chapter 5, 'Symptom relief for advanced heart failure'. In the very terminal stages of heart failure, usually only diuretics are continued. These can be administered orally or by a continuous subcutaneous infusion if intravenous access is difficult or deemed inappropriate. If tolerated, digoxin is sometimes continued to slow heart rate and improve symptoms without affecting blood pressure. Rationalisation of medication in patients who are dying is discussed in Chapter 8, 'Care of the patient dying from heart failure'.

DEVICE THERAPY IN ADVANCED DISEASE AND APPROACHING END OF LIFE

In very advanced heart failure and as end of life approaches, it is important to consider deactivation of an ICD or CRT-D device. In general terms, continuation of the pacing function of these devices will be appropriate. CRT pacing will provide ongoing benefit with respect to symptoms of fatigue and dyspnoea and will reduce the risk of cardiac decompensation and hospital admission. Often, the pacing function of a CRT-D or an ICD will be necessary to prevent recurrent symptomatic bradyarrhythmia. Neither CRT pacing nor pacing via an ICD will prolong life or cause any pain or distress in the terminal stages, and patients and their families should be reassured of this.

Towards end of life, deactivation of the defibrillator function of a CRT-D device or ICD is very often appropriate and in the best interests of the patient. As end of life approaches, patients with heart failure may be prone to unstable ventricular rhythms causing recurrent shocks with marked associated pain and distress.[51] Discussions regarding disabling the defibrillator function of a device should be prospective and tailored to the individual patient dependent on their clinical status, arrhythmia burden and experience of previous device therapies. Patients may have unrealistic expectations of successful ICD defibrillation based on previous experience from earlier in their disease trajectory. They may also have significant unrecognised misconceptions about how their device works and may even anticipate instantaneous death on deactivation of the defibrillator.[52] Therefore, the concept of device deactivation must be conveyed sensitively to patients and their carers. Usually, these discussions form a part of anticipatory care planning, along with consideration of the appropriateness of other interventions towards end of life, such as cardiopulmonary resuscitation (CPR). It is important to recognise that while defibrillator deactivation is often consistent with a 'do not attempt cardiopulmonary resuscitation' (DNACPR) order, the two are not mutually exclusive. For example, a patient may have a chronic illness and be experiencing difficulties with their device with inappropriate shocks. In that situation, deactivation of the defibrillator is indicated, but attempted CPR may still be entirely appropriate. Another example would be a patient for who a DNACPR order would be appropriate due to anticipated futility in the context of a cardiopulmonary arrest, but continuing active implantable defibrillator function would still be reasonable to treat isolated malignant arrhythmias. The appropriateness of a patient's defibrillator device remaining active should be regularly considered throughout the disease trajectory by all healthcare professionals involved. Any discussion regarding device deactivation should prompt discussion regarding CPR and vice versa. More detail regarding device therapy at the end of life is given in Chapter 8.

REFERENCES

1 Faris R, Flather MD, Purcell H *et al.* Diuretics for heart failure. *Cochrane Database Syst Rev.* 2006; (1): CD003838.
2 Acute Infarction Ramipril Efficacy (AIRE) Study Investigators. Effect of ramipril on mortality and morbidity of survivors of acute myocardial infarction with clinical evidence of heart failure. *Lancet.* 1993; **342**(8875): 821–8.
3 Cooperative North Scandinavian Enalapril Survival Study (CONSENSUS) Trial Study Group. Effects of enalapril on mortality in severe congestive heart failure. Results of the Cooperative North Scandinavian Enalapril Survival Study (CONSENSUS). *N Engl J Med.* 1987; **316**(23): 1429–35.
4 Studies of Left Ventricular Dysfunction (SOLVD) Investigators. Effect of enalapril on survival in patients with reduced left ventricular ejection fractions and congestive heart failure. *N Engl J Med.* 1991; **325**(5): 293–302.
5 Pfeffer MA, Braunwald E, Moyé LA *et al.* Effect of captopril on mortality and morbidity in patients with left ventricular dysfunction after myocardial infarction. Results of the survival and ventricular enlargement trial. The SAVE Investigators. *N Engl J Med.* 1992; **327**(10): 669–77.
6 Packer M, Poole-Wilson PA, Armstrong PW *et al.* Comparative effects of low and high doses of the angiotensin-converting enzyme inhibitor, lisinopril, on morbidity and mortality in chronic heart failure. ATLAS Study Group. *Circulation.* 1999; **100**(23): 2312–18.
7 Torp-Pedersen C, Køber L. Effect of ACE inhibitor trandolapril on life expectancy of patients with reduced left-ventricular function after acute myocardial infarction. TRACE Study Group. Trandolapril Cardiac Evaluation. *Lancet.* 1999; **354**(9172): 9–12.
8 Jessup M, Brozena S. Heart failure. *N Engl J Med.* 2003; **348**(20): 2007–18.
9 McMurray JJ, Adamopoulos S, Anker SD *et al.* ESC guidelines for the diagnosis and treatment of acute and chronic heart failure 2012: The Task Force for the Diagnosis

and Treatment of Acute and Chronic Heart Failure 2012 of the European Society of Cardiology. Developed in collaboration with the Heart Failure Association (HFA) of the ESC. *Eur Heart J*. 2012; **33**(14): 1787–847.

10 Metra M, Dei Cas L, Massie BM. Treatment of heart failure in the elderly: never say it's too late. *Eur Heart J*. 2009; **30**(4): 391–3.

11 Flather MD, Yusuf S, Køber L *et al*. Long-term ACE-inhibitor therapy in patients with heart failure or left-ventricular dysfunction: a systematic overview of data from individual patients. ACE-Inhibitor Myocardial Infarction Collaborative Group. *Lancet*. 2000; **355**(9215): 1575–81.

12 Granger CB, McMurray JJ, Yusuf S *et al*. Effects of candesartan in patients with chronic heart failure and reduced left-ventricular systolic function intolerant to angiotensin-converting-enzyme inhibitors: the CHARM-Alternative trial. *Lancet*. 2003; **362**(9386): 772–6.

13 Pitt B, Poole-Wilson PA, Segal R *et al*. Effect of losartan compared with captopril on mortality in patients with symptomatic heart failure: randomised trial – the Losartan Heart Failure Survival Study ELITE II. *Lancet*. 2000; **355**(9215): 1582–7.

14 Pitt B, Segal R, Martinez FA *et al*. Randomized trial of losartan versus captopril in patients over 65 with heart failure (Evaluation of Losartan in the Elderly Study, ELITE). *Lancet*. 1997; **349**(9054): 747–52.

15 Cohn JN, Tognoni G. A randomized trial of the angiotensin-receptor blocker valsartan in chronic heart failure. *N Engl J Med*. 2001; **345**(23): 1667–75.

16 McMurray JJ, Ostergren J, Swedberg K *et al*. Effects of candesartan in patients with chronic heart failure and reduced left-ventricular systolic function taking angiotensin-converting-enzyme inhibitors: the CHARM-Added trial. *Lancet*. 2003; **362**(9386): 767–71.

17 Baruch L, Glazer RD, Aknay N *et al*. Morbidity, mortality, physiologic and functional parameters in elderly and non-elderly patients in the Valsartan Heart Failure Trial (Val-HeFT). *Am Heart J*. 2004; **148**(6): 951–7.

18 Cohn JN, Archibald DG, Ziesche S *et al*. Effect of vasodilator therapy on mortality in chronic congestive heart failure. Results of a Veterans Administration Cooperative Study. *N Engl J Med*. 1986; **314**(24): 1547–52.

19 Cohn JN, Johnson G, Ziesche S *et al*. A comparison of enalapril with hydralazine-isosorbide dinitrate in the treatment of chronic congestive heart failure. *N Engl J Med*. 1991; **325**(5): 303–10.

20 Taylor AL, Ziesche S, Yancy C *et al*. Combination of isosorbide dinitrate and hydralazine in blacks with heart failure. *N Engl J Med*. 2004; **351**(20): 2049–57.

21 Cardiac Insufficiency Bisoprolol Study (CIBIS) Investigators and Committees. A randomized trial of beta-blockade in heart failure. The Cardiac Insufficiency Bisoprolol Study (CIBIS). *Circulation*. 1994; **90**(4): 1765–73.

22 CIBIS-II Investigators and Committees. The Cardiac Insufficiency Bisoprolol Study II (CIBIS-II): a randomised trial. *Lancet*. 1999; **353**(9146): 9–13.

23 Colucci WS, Packer M, Bristow MR *et al*. Carvedilol inhibits clinical progression in patients with mild symptoms of heart failure. US Carvedilol Heart Failure Study Group. *Circulation*. 1996; **94**(11): 2800–6.

24 Packer M, Coats AJ, Fowler MB *et al*. Effect of carvedilol on survival in severe chronic heart failure. *N Engl J Med*. 2001; **344**(22): 1651–8.

25 Metoprolol CR/XL Randomised Intervention Trial in Congestive Heart Failure (MERIT-HF) Study Group. Effect of metoprolol CR/XL in chronic heart failure: Metoprolol CR/XL Randomised Intervention Trial in Congestive Heart Failure (MERIT-HF). *Lancet.* 1999; **353**(9169): 2001–7.

26 Kotecha D, Holmes J, Krum H *et al.* Efficacy of β blockers in patients with heart failure plus atrial fibrillation: an individual-patient data meta-analysis. *Lancet.* 2014; **384**(9961): 2235–43.

27 Dulin BR, Haas SJ, Abraham WT *et al.* Do elderly systolic heart failure patients benefit from beta blockers to the same extent as the non-elderly? Meta-analysis of >12 000 patients in large-scale clinical trials. *Am J Cardiol.* 2005; **95**(7): 896–8.

28 Flather MD, Shibata MC, Coats AJ *et al.* Randomized trial to determine the effect of nebivolol on mortality and cardiovascular hospital admission in elderly patients with heart failure (SENIORS). *Eur Heart J.* 2005; **26**(3): 215–25.

29 Pitt B, Zannad F, Remme WJ *et al.* The effect of spironolactone on morbidity and mortality in patients with severe heart failure. Randomized Aldactone Evaluation Study Investigators. *N Engl J Med.* 1999; **341**(10): 709–17.

30 Zannad F, McMurray JJ, Krum H *et al.* Eplerenone in patients with systolic heart failure and mild symptoms. *N Engl J Med.* 2011; **364**(1): 11–21.

31 Pitt B, Remme W, Zannad F *et al.* Eplerenone, a selective aldosterone blocker, in patients with left ventricular dysfunction after myocardial infarction. *N Engl J Med.* 2003; **348**(14): 1309–21.

32 Rich MW. Office management of heart failure in the elderly. *Am J Med.* 2005; **118**(4): 342–8.

33 Digitalis Investigation Group. The effect of digoxin on mortality and morbidity in patients with heart failure. *N Engl J Med.* 1997; **336**(8): 525–33.

34 Rathore SS, Curtis JP, Wang Y *et al.* Association of serum digoxin concentration and outcomes in patients with heart failure. *JAMA.* 2003; **289**(7): 871–8.

35 Anter E, Jessup M, Callans DJ. Atrial fibrillation and heart failure: treatment considerations for a dual epidemic. *Circulation.* 2009 May 12; **119**(18): 2516-25.

36 Shah M, Avgil Tsadok M, Jackevicius CA *et al.* Relation of digoxin use in atrial fibrillation and the risk of all-cause mortality in patients ≥65 years of age with versus without heart failure. *Am J Cardiol.* 2014; **114**(3): 401–6.

37 Rich MW, McSherry F, Williford WO *et al.* Effect of age on mortality, hospitalizations and response to digoxin in patients with heart failure: the DIG study. *J Am Coll Cardiol.* 2001; **38**(3): 806–13.

38 Swedberg K, Komajda M, Böhm M *et al.* Ivabradine and outcomes in chronic heart failure (SHIFT): a randomised placebo-controlled study. *Lancet.* 2010; **376**(9744): 875–85.

39 Stulc T, Ceška R. Ivabradine, coronary heart disease, and heart failure: time for reappraisal. *Curr Atheroscler Rep.* 2014; **16**(12): 463.

40 Homma S, Thompson JL, Pullicino PM *et al.* Warfarin and aspirin in patients with heart failure and sinus rhythm. *N Engl J Med.* 2012; **366**(20): 1859–69.

41 Cleland JG, Daubert JC, Erdmann E *et al.* The effect of cardiac resynchronization on morbidity and mortality in heart failure. *N Engl J Med.* 2005; **352**(15): 1539–49.

42 Moss AJ, Hall WJ, Cannom DS *et al.* Cardiac-resynchronization therapy for the prevention of heart-failure events. *N Engl J Med.* 2009; **361**(14): 1329–38.

43 Tang AS, Wells GA, Talajic M *et al.* Cardiac-resynchronization therapy for mild-to-moderate heart failure. *N Engl J Med.* 2010; **363**(25): 2385–95.

44 Curtis AB, Worley SJ, Adamson PB *et al.* Biventricular pacing for atrioventricular block and systolic dysfunction. *N Engl J Med.* 2013; **368**(17): 1585–93.

45 Chung ES, Leon AR, Tavazzi L *et al.* Results of the Predictors of Response to CRT (PROSPECT) trial. *Circulation.* 2008; **117**(20): 2608–16.

46 Antiarrhythmics versus Implantable Defibrillators (AVID) Investigators. A comparison of antiarrhythmic-drug therapy with implantable defibrillators in patients resuscitated from near-fatal ventricular arrhythmias. *N Engl J Med.* 1997; **337**(22): 1576–83.

47 Moss AJ, Zareba W, Hall WJ *et al.* Prophylactic implantation of a defibrillator in patients with myocardial infarction and reduced ejection fraction. *N Engl J Med.* 2002; **346**(12): 877–83.

48 Bardy GH, Lee KL, Mark DB *et al.* Amiodarone or an implantable cardioverter-defibrillator for congestive heart failure. *N Engl J Med.* 2005; **352**(3): 225–37.

49 Rose EA, Gelijns AC, Moskowitz AJ *et al.* Long-term use of a left ventricular assist device for end-stage heart failure. *N Engl J Med.* 2001; **345**(20): 1435–43.

50 Slaughter MS, Rogers JG, Milano CA *et al.* Advanced heart failure treated with continuous-flow left ventricular assist device. *N Engl J Med.* 2009; **361**(23): 2241–51.

51 Kinch Westerdahl A, Sjöblom J, Mattiasson AC *et al.* Implantable cardioverter-defibrillator therapy before death: high risk for painful shocks at end of life. *Circulation.* 2014; **129**(4): 422–9.

52 Strömberg A, Fluur C, Miller J *et al.* ICD recipients' understanding of ethical issues, ICD function, and practical consequences of withdrawing the ICD in the end-of-life. *Pacing Clin Electrophysiol.* 2014; **37**(7): 834–42.

CHAPTER 4

Prognosis in advanced heart failure

RICHARD LEHMAN AND AMY GADOUD

INTRODUCTION

In Chapter 1, 'The need for palliative care in heart failure', we noted the often-erratic disease trajectory of heart failure and the frequency of sudden death – factors that would seem to make prediction in individual patients very difficult. The rather scanty data we have about doctors' predictions in heart failure would seem to bear this out. In early heart failure, primary care doctors may tend to overestimate the risk of death – at least in Switzerland.[1] In contrast, the Study to Understand Prognoses and Preferences for Outcomes and Risks of Treatments (SUPPORT),[2] carried out in the mid-1990s in the USA, found that 50% of heart failure patients were given a prognosis of more than 6 months on the day before they died. Moreover, clinicians failed to act on prognostic information that was available; patients continued to receive futile treatment, and experienced poor quality of life and care at the end of life. Clinicians not only require prognostic information but also the judgement and courage to use it appropriately.[3]

Here, we will look at some of the numerous factors that have been identified as helping to predict prognosis. There are hundreds in the literature. For example, a narrative review of prognostic variables in heart failure identified over 300 proposed prognostic variables for heart failure,[4] and new prognostic variables for heart failure are being discovered almost continuously.[5] However, many of these are not clinically useful or have little evidence to support them. For those that have been more thoroughly investigated, they are often adjusted for by different covariates, so cannot be combined in a meta-analysis or compared to identify the relative strength of different predictors.

In this chapter, we concentrate on those prognostic variables that are robust and easy to apply in a clinical context. There is no easily accessible review of prognosis in heart failure from the perspective of palliative care, so this chapter tries to deal with the whole picture, as well as with the specific tests and scoring systems that are of most use in predicting death in individual patients with advanced disease.

Throughout most of this section, we try to use data from studies done on large series of patients to refine our predictions about the individual patient in front of us. The purpose of this chapter is to help you determine more accurately which patients are likely to have a poor prognosis – for example, those who may be in their last year of life – although it should be noted that this time frame should not be a way of excluding access to palliative care for people with palliative care needs who appear to have a better prognosis, at least, in terms of time.

THE EVIDENCE BASE FOR PROGNOSIS
Challenges with prognostic study design

It has been said that prognostic models are easy to produce, hard to validate, harder still to implement in clinical practice and evidence of impact on decision-making is nearly always lacking.[6] The model or prognostic variable should be validated in other populations.[6,7] However, not only is it necessary for a prognostic tool to be valid, but the effect on clinical practice should also be demonstrated.[8]

The measured outcome requires careful thought. Mode of death (e.g. sudden or progressive) – appropriately defined and preferably independently confirmed – may be useful; however, mortality may not be the most important outcome to patients;[6] others, such as symptoms or quality of life, may be more important. Prognosis is not just about death, and the prediction of worsening of symptoms or need for additional care support may be useful for both patients and professionals.

WHAT DO WE KNOW?

Our knowledge of what determines outcome in heart failure comes from a number of sources. First, there are studies based in the community[9–12] that follow up a large number of patients identified as having heart failure. Such studies have the great advantage of looking at a typical population with heart failure. As diagnostic criteria vary and disease registers may not be wholly accurate, such studies may be difficult to compare accurately, but they are still the most useful guide to what happens in primary care.

Second, there are studies based wholly or partly on the follow-up of patients after a hospital admission for heart failure. Although these studies do not give an accurate picture of overall prognosis for all classes of heart failure in the community, they are still very useful in our quest for indicators of adverse outlook in individual patients. The Hillingdon study[13] can be included among these, because although it did its best to encourage direct recruitment from primary care, it ended up with a cohort drawn largely from hospital admissions for heart failure.

Third, there are data from the large interventional studies, such as those that established the role of angiotensin-converting enzyme inhibitors and beta-adrenergic blockers in the past two decades. Unfortunately, the largest and best-known studies recruited from hospital populations are not comparable to the patients we typically encounter in the community – they were predominantly male, younger than average and usually selected for the absence of some kinds of co-morbidity. The Candesartan in Heart Failure: Assessment of Reduction in Mortality and Morbidity (CHARM) study[14] of 7599 patients (69% male, mean age 66 years) has been very thoroughly analysed and is perhaps the best source of a risk score derived from history and common clinical variables, including cardiac, but not biochemical, investigations.

Lastly, and least typically, are patients undergoing selection for cardiac transplantation. They are mostly younger people with cardiomyopathy or very severe ischaemic damage. They are the most intensively studied group, and there is an extensive literature on physiological indicators that predict their likelihood of death.[15-17] However, only fragments of this knowledge can be usefully applied to the patients we typically see in everyday clinical practice.

GENERAL INDICATORS OF PROGNOSIS

General, easily assessed clinical features give us an idea of how our patient is likely to fare and are discussed here first. Later, we will look at more sophisticated tests and scores.

Age

In the Rotterdam whole-population study,[9] the average age of heart failure patients was 77 years, and, over 5 years, their risk of death was 41% – a much lower mortality than in most hospital-recruited studies but well above that in the age-matched population without heart failure, which was 15%. Every 10 years of age doubles the likelihood of death within 4 years in patients with heart failure. The Olmsted County study,[10] carried out at the same time in the USA, found exactly the same age distribution but a worse 5-year prognosis (overall case-fatality, 67%).

Hospital admission

In the Ontario study of patients discharged after a first admission for heart failure, case-fatality rates were much higher than in general population-based studies, at 40.1% at 12 months (rather than 5 years) in those over 75 years. For patients under 50 years, it was 13.5%. In the Hillingdon study,[13] in which 82% of the study population had been admitted to hospital for a first episode of heart failure, the overall case-fatality rate was similar, at 38% after 12 months.

It seems that heart failure sufficiently severe to warrant hospital admission has a much worse outlook than heart failure that can be managed entirely in primary care. Analysis of the CHARM randomised controlled trial also demonstrated hospitalisation was a statistically significant predictor of mortality, but its effects reduced over time since admission.[18]

Gender

Women with a diagnosis of heart failure generally live longer than men: in one study (Cardiac Insufficiency Bisoprolol Study [CIBIS]-II),[19] the difference in mortality was 36%, although this may not be true of heart failure due to ischaemic heart disease. A cohort study of hospitalised patients in the USA aged from 35 to 84 also showed a survival advantage for women with heart failure.[20]

The Meta-Analysis Global Group in Chronic Heart Failure (MAGGIC) individual patient data meta-analysis demonstrated that survival is better for women with heart failure than for men with heart failure, irrespective of ejection fraction (EF). This survival benefit is slightly more marked in non-ischaemic heart failure but is attenuated by concomitant diabetes.[21]

Aetiology

The aetiology of heart failure is changing with time, as rheumatic valvular disease is becoming rare, ischaemic heart disease is decreasing and more people are being diagnosed with heart failure and preserved ejection fraction. Moreover, most patients with heart failure are now receiving drug therapy that prolongs life, so data like those from Framingham between 1948 and 1988[22] are now of purely historical value. Even the more recent Framingham data (1989–99)[11] may be misleading in the context of rapidly changing patterns of cardiovascular morbidity and therapy.

In general, however, the studies show that, currently, heart failure due to known ischaemic disease has the worst prognosis. Yet, infiltrative causes such as amyloidosis have an even worse prognosis.[23]

CO-MORBIDITY

Most patients with heart failure have other problems of old age, and these can markedly affect prognosis. Some of these co-morbidities may be due, at least in part, to the heart failure itself – this is probably true of depression, anaemia and cognitive impairment. Co-morbidities can be grouped together in scoring systems such as the Charlson Comorbidity Index, with twice the mortality in the highest scoring group as those in the group with a score of zero.

Diabetes

In community studies of heart failure, diabetes (mostly type 2) is typically found in 10%–20% of patients. The data on the prognostic influence of diabetes are conflicting. Most studies find that diabetes has an adverse prognostic effect, and this is certainly true of heart failure accompanied by systolic dysfunction.[24] However, diabetes can also be associated with diastolic heart failure, which has a better prognosis. The wide disparity between the various studies of prognosis in heart failure accompanied by diabetes may be explained by differences in case definition, stage of disease and ethnic mix.

Osteoarthritis

With the average age of heart failure patients in the late 70s, the majority of heart failure patients are likely to have some degree of osteoarthritis. This features as an adverse prognostic factor in a large study from Toronto,[25] perhaps because these patients are more likely to be prescribed non-steroidal anti-inflammatory drugs, which become more dangerous as heart failure worsens and renal function declines.

Depression

Depression is common in heart failure and, in its later stages, may be directly linked to cytokine release, causing depletion of serotonin. It is a markedly adverse prognostic factor,[26] but one which can probably be ameliorated by serotonin reuptake inhibitors.

Anaemia

Anaemia is a common precipitant of clinical heart failure and often responds initially to iron supplementation. However, when heart failure progresses and renal impairment increases, erythropoietin production declines, leading to anaemia, which worsens breathlessness, impairs tissue oxygenation and is refractory to treatment. Thus, anaemia becomes an increasingly adverse prognostic feature as heart failure worsens.[27]

Cognitive impairment

In heart failure, cognitive impairment is common[28] and markedly worsens outlook,[29] even outscoring cancer in some series. This may reflect a number of factors: dementia itself is linked with high mortality independently of heart disease and patients with dementia may receive less intensive treatment and are likely to be less compliant with complex drug regimens. In some cases, apparent cognitive impairment may be directly due to depression – the 'depressive pseudodementia' syndrome. In end-stage heart failure, cognitive impairment may be due to complex factors affecting brain oxygenation, including anaemia, reduced cerebral blood supply and disordered breathing.

Pulmonary disease

Pulmonary disease is very common in older patients with heart failure, many of who have smoked for most of their lives. Respiratory infection is also a common cause of decompensation and hospital admission in heart failure. These aspects, added to the fact that heart failure is fundamentally a syndrome of impaired tissue oxygenation, make it remarkable that respiratory disease is not a more strongly adverse prognostic feature.

Cancer

Inevitably, many older patients will have cancer as well as heart failure. To group all cancers together as 'malignancy', as in some studies, is of interest only to those looking at the approximate disease burden in the population. Each patient with cancer and heart failure will have an individual prognostic picture, as well as individual and complex needs.

Atrial fibrillation

Atrial fibrillation (AF) is common in heart failure, and new-onset AF often leads to sudden decompensation of previously stable heart failure. If this happens, the prognosis immediately worsens.[30] However, in general, the observed higher mortality in patients with heart failure and AF seems to be related to other prognostic factors associated with AF; that is, it is not independently associated with a poor prognosis.[31]

FUNCTIONAL INDICATORS

Remarkably, the patients with heart failure who are likely to survive longest are those we might think at highest risk – those who are overweight, have high blood pressure, high cholesterol and drink alcohol. This has been labelled 'reverse epidemiology'.[32] So it is worth going through some of the data on various indicators of function in these patients, because it is not necessarily simply a matter of common sense.

Renal impairment

'Renal disease' is often listed as a co-morbidity in heart failure, but it is perhaps more helpful to regard it as an intrinsic functional consequence of advanced heart failure.[33] The physiological response to heart failure is, to an important extent, a response to decreased renal perfusion, but, as we have seen in Chapter 2, the response actually worsens the problem and leads to the so-called 'cardio-renal syndrome', a vicious spiral of combined heart and kidney failure.

Of course, there may be other factors that worsen renal function. These include obstructive nephropathy in older men with prostatism, diabetic nephropathy and renal artery disease. Many of the drugs given for heart failure can worsen renal function initially and lead to a rise in creatinine and a fall in sodium (*see* 'Sodium' in the 'Specific markers' section, p. 68).

Blood pressure

Most people with heart failure have a history of elevated blood pressure at some stage in their lives. Nevertheless, a damaged heart cannot maintain high pressures; and, further, all treatment for heart failure lowers blood pressure. So, too, does the release of natriuretic peptides from overstretched atria and ventricles. Thus, once heart failure has set in, a low blood pressure is a marker for worsening disease and is associated with a poor prognosis.

Weight

Weight loss of more than 7.5% of previous normal weight over 6 months or more is associated with a very poor prognosis in heart failure.[34] This is the syndrome of cardiac cachexia, which is very similar to the cachexia of advanced cancer and, in common with it, is probably driven by cytokines. However, even if we remove bias by excluding any distorting effect from cardiac cachexia, there is still a generally favourable association between weight and survival in heart failure that extends well into the range usually labelled 'obese'. This is often described as an 'obesity paradox': decreased survival in lower body mass index but increased survival in higher body mass index.[14,35,36]

Exercise capacity

Exercise capacity in heart failure shows little relation to systolic EF but is linked to prognosis. This extends all the way from maximal exercise on a treadmill to pedometer measurements obtained from people who can barely walk. Some measurement techniques are discussed following. Exercise training can improve quality of life and health status in patients with heart failure.[37,38]

Diuretic resistance

As part of the cardio-renal syndrome, patients become less responsive to loop diuretics, or patchily responsive, so that they alternate between hypovolaemia and fluid overload. One retrospective analysis of an interventional trial has attempted to quantify diuretic response in relation to prognosis.[39] In normal clinical practice, the best way to evaluate response is by trial of treatment and daily weighing: patients who need constant adjustment of their diuretics certainly have a poorer outlook.

Abnormal breathing

Heart failure is a state of chemoreceptor overdrive, so that patterns of respiration are abnormally sensitive to fluctuations in oxygen (O_2) and carbon dioxide, and, as a result, breathing is inappropriately effortful. There is some evidence that reducing this overdrive using opioids is not only symptomatically beneficial but may also be functionally beneficial, too.

Many patients with heart failure exhibit an apnoeic (Cheyne–Stokes) pattern of breathing at night, which is of little prognostic importance. However, Cheyne–Stokes breathing by day predicts death within a few months.[40]

PHYSIOLOGICAL MEASUREMENTS

Most physiological testing in heart failure is done in specialist units, usually either for research or for refining prognosis in younger patients who are being considered for surgery, including transplantation or left ventricular assist devices. The following are some of the prognostically useful measurements.

Peak O_2 uptake

The heart is required to produce a supply of oxygenated blood to all body systems under all normal conditions, including normal exertion. One way to measure how well the heart is functioning is to measure how much O_2 a patient can use up when exercising to the limit of their capacity. Until recently, this has been considered the gold standard for prognosis, especially when used sequentially;[41] however, it requires highly specialised laboratory equipment and is, therefore, only normally used in research and in the evaluation of younger patients for surgery or transplantation.

Peak exercise cardiac power output

This test comes close to the gold standard for determining the degree of physiological heart failure, but it is not widely available. It consists of measurements of cardiac output using carbon-dioxide re-breathing techniques, and the cardiac output is then multiplied by the mean arterial blood pressure to give the cardiac power output.[23]

Daily activity level

At the opposite extreme from these complex laboratory-based measurements of 'pure' physiological parameters is to use a simple instrument to measure what patients actually do in their everyday lives. One method is to attach a pedometer to measure the weekly walking distance. This is a powerful prognostic tool,[42] with the shorter the distance walked – such as in a 6-minute walk test (6MWT) – the greater the risk of death.[43] American Thoracic Society Guidelines (2002) recommend the use of the 6MWT not only in subjects with lung disease but also in those with heart failure as a one-time measure of functional status and for the evaluation of the effects of therapy and prognostic stratification.[44]

Activities of daily living

A simple assessment of the degree to which heart failure affects the activities of daily living (ADLs) has been shown to have prognostic value in a study of a typical older heart failure population in the USA.[45] Difficulty with nine ADLs was assessed by questionnaire and patients were divided into three categories of ADL difficulty (no/minimal, moderate, severe). Mortality increased with increasing ADL difficulty; the hazard ratio (95% confidence interval) for death was 1.49 (1.22–1.82) and 2.26 (1.79–2.86) for those with moderate and severe difficulty, respectively, compared with those with no/minimal difficulty. This suggests that a very basic holistic assessment of heart failure patients may provide most of the information needed to determine both prognosis and the need for supportive care.

Heart rate variability

As heart failure progresses, there is increasing autonomic dysfunction. This leads to a diminution in the ability of the cardiovascular system to accommodate to changing demands and can be measured in several ways. The simplest way is to do a 24-hour ambulatory electrocardiogram (ECG) and perform an automated analysis for heart rate variability. Patients at high risk of death from progressive heart failure[46] show the least heart rate variability, and this is also true for sudden death.[47,48]

Electrocardiographic changes

Almost all patients with heart failure have ECG abnormalities, and many detailed features of the ECG have been looked at for their prognostic significance. However, Q waves and AF are probably the only simple and widely available ECG parameters that clinicians use to help prediction in daily practice. Nevertheless, it should be remembered that these studies were conducted before the widespread use of implantable cardiovertor defibrillator / biventricular pacemakers and beta-blockers, which have reduced sudden death.

Restrictive filling pattern (echocardiographic)

Over recent years, there has been increasing interest in impaired ventricular filling as a contributor to heart failure syndrome. Various methods of measurement have been proposed, and some of these are now robust enough to become part of routine echocardiographic assessment in patients with heart failure.

A restrictive filling pattern on Doppler echo is more closely related to prognosis than a decreased systolic EF.[49]

Systolic EF

The measurement of the proportion of blood pumped out by the ventricle at each beat (left ventricular systolic ejection fraction [LVSF]) was used as the entry criterion for nearly all interventional heart failure trials from 1980 onwards, and this has bedevilled the subject ever since. It means that our evidence base is largely for heart failure with reduced LVSF, even though the LVSF has less predictive value than most parameters discussed in this section. However, it is reasonably easy to measure by various means, the least accurate of which is echocardiography, and it has some overall prognostic value.[50]

The major trials in patients with heart failure mainly enrolled patients with an EF of less than 35%, and, to date, it is only in these patients that effective therapies have been demonstrated. More recently, another group of heart failure patients has been described: those with an EF of between 40% and 45% and no other causal cardiac abnormality. Some of these patients do not have an entirely normal EF (generally considered to be >50%), but, in addition, do not have a major reduction in systolic function either. Because of this, the term 'heart failure with preserved ejection fraction' was coined to describe these patients. Most have evidence of diastolic dysfunction, which is generally accepted as the likely cause of heart failure in these patients (hence the term 'diastolic heart failure'). However, more sensitive measures of systolic function may show abnormalities in patients with a preserved or even normal EF – thus the preference for stating preserved or reduced EF over preserved or reduced systolic function.[51] Patients with heart failure with preserved ejection fraction have a worse prognosis than those with a reduced EF.[52]

SPECIFIC MARKERS

Blood urea nitrogen/Creatinine/Uric acid

As part of heart failure syndrome, renal perfusion declines and neurohormonal overdrive ensues. As a result, the ability of the kidney to excrete nitrogenous waste products becomes impaired, and the plasma level of all these products – urea, uric acid and creatinine – goes up. In advanced heart failure, there is also extra production of nitrogenous breakdown products from muscle catabolism. Studies of individual nitrogenous products such as uric acid[53] and total blood urea nitrogen[54] have shown that increasing blood levels are associated with worsening prognosis. As a single variable, the predictor serum creatinine had the highest sensitivity and specificity for predicting death at 12 months.[12] Other multivariable models are available but have not been externally validated.[55–8]

Cystatin C

Nitrogenous waste products are not a very accurate indicator of renal function, and there has been recent interest in markers that correlate more closely to glomerular filtration rate. A promising candidate, not yet available for routine clinical use, is cystatin C, a protein continuously produced at a steady rate and freely filtered by the glomerulus. Serum levels of cystatin C have been shown to reflect glomerular filtration rate much more accurately than serum or plasma levels of creatinine. In a recent study, levels of cystatin C in patients with heart failure predicted cardiac events even in those with normal creatinine levels.[59]

Sodium

As heart failure worsens, the level of sodium in the blood falls for two reasons: the first is the ever-increasing release of natriuretic (i.e. sodium-expelling) hormones from the heart, and the second is the increasing need to use sodium-depleting diuretics to relieve symptoms in advanced heart failure. Thus, a fall in plasma sodium is a very useful and universally available surrogate measure for worsening heart failure.[60]

Troponins

One of the most significant advances in cardiology over the past decade has been the rapid adoption of cardiac troponin measurement as a way of detecting myocardial damage in acute coronary syndromes. The troponins are only released if there is myocardial cell injury, and we saw in Chapter 2 ('Cell death', p. 27) that myocytes are injured in advanced heart failure and die in one of two ways – necrosis, which is usually due to acute ischaemia, or apoptosis, which can be caused by a number of mechanisms. In fact, there is probably an overlap between these mechanisms, and both may result in troponin release. In other words, troponin levels reflect a process of actual myocyte damage and loss in advanced heart failure. They are therefore of important prognostic value,[61] and troponin measurements are now routinely available in all acute hospitals. Persistently elevated troponin levels are associated with an adverse prognosis. However, they add only modestly to risk discrimination and do not improve calibration of risk models. Routine assessment of troponin concentrations in chronic heart failure patients is not currently recommended.[62,63]

B-type natriuretic peptide

B-type, or 'brain', natriuretic peptide (BNP) is a potent hormone released by the ventricular myocytes in response to stretch or inflammation. Since heart failure involves both stretch and inflammation, it is impossible to have uncompensated heart failure without an elevation of BNP. The word 'natriuretic' simply means 'promoting salt and water excretion', and we have seen earlier in this chapter that falling sodium can be used as a measure of hormonal activation in advancing heart failure. So, why not measure BNP directly? There are several ways of doing this, and whichever assay is chosen, the prognostic power is impressive – in fact, greater than complex scoring systems based on the physiological parameters detailed earlier.[64] If we combine BNP with troponins, we can get even more predictive information.[62,63] Thus, when it is available, BNP is the most useful measure of progression in heart failure and predicts both progressive heart failure[65] and sudden death.[66] However, only serial measurements would provide a clear picture of progression.

SCORING SYSTEMS FOR PROGNOSIS

We have seen that there are numerous factors that a clinician can use to assess which patients with heart failure may be getting closer to death. Of the biochemical markers, BNP (or N-terminal pro-brain natriuretic peptide) shows outstanding promise as part of a validated score. There are a variety of such scores in heart failure, ranging from the New York Heart Association (NYHA) classification, which is just a simple grading by breathlessness and fatigue, to the very complex multifactorial scores used in heart transplantation clinics, such as the heart failure survival score (HFSS) or German Transplant Society (GTS) score.[67]

Minnesota Living with Heart Failure Questionnaire

As its name implies, this questionnaire was designed as a measurement tool for quality of life in heart failure and has been confirmed valuable in many studies for over a decade.[68] It has proved of prognostic value alongside BNP[69] and in addition to the Utrecht and Epidémiologie de l'Insuffisance Cardiaque Avancée en Lorraine (EPICAL) scores, of which details are given following.

Enhanced Feedback for Effective Cardiac Treatment (EFFECT)

The EFFECT study[25] was carried out in exemplary fashion by investigators based in Toronto who studied two cohorts of patients following a hospital admission for heart failure to generate and validate a prognostic scoring system based on that presented in Table 4.1. The predictive usefulness of the EFFECT scoring system is demonstrated in Figure 4.1. It has been validated more recently in a prospective cohort of patients after index hospitalisation for heart failure.[39]

An online calculator is available ([www.ccort.ca/Research/CHFRiskModel.](www.ccort.ca/Research/CHFRiskModel.aspx) [aspx](www.ccort.ca/Research/CHFRiskModel.aspx) [accessed 18 May 2015]). However, this does not include BNP and was determined prior to the widespread use of the modern medical management of heart failure with beta-blockers, angiotensin-converting enzyme I and so on.

TABLE 4.1 Heart failure risk scoring system from the Enhanced Feedback for Effective Cardiac Treatment (EFFECT) study*

Variable	Number of points	
	30-day score[†]	1-year score[‡]
Years	+ age (in years)	+ age (in years)
Respiratory rate, min (minimum 20; maximum 45)[§]	+ rate (in breaths/min)	+ rate (in breaths/min)
Systolic blood pressure (mmHg)[¶]		
≥180	−60	−50
160–79	−55	−45
140–59	−50	−40
120–39	−45	−35
100–19	−40	−30
90–99	−35	−25
<90	−30	−20
Urea nitrogen (maximum, 60 mg/dL)[§**]	+ level (in mg/dL)	+ level (in mg/dL)
Sodium concentration <136 mEq/L	+10	+10
Cerebrovascular disease	+10	+10
Dementia	+20	+15
Chronic obstructive pulmonary disease	+10	+10
Hepatic cirrhosis	+25	+35
Cancer	+15	+15
Haemoglobin <10.0 g/dL (<100 g/L)	NA	+10

Notes: *An electronic version of the risk scoring system is available at: [www.ccort.ca/Research/CHFRiskModel.](www.ccort.ca/Research/CHFRiskModel.aspx) [aspx](www.ccort.ca/Research/CHFRiskModel.aspx) (accessed 18 May 2015). [†]Calculated as age + respiratory rate + systolic blood pressure + urea nitrogen + sodium points + cerebrovascular disease points + dementia points + chronic obstructive pulmonary disease points + hepatic cirrhosis points + cancer points. [‡]Calculated as age + respiratory rate + systolic blood pressure + urea nitrogen + sodium points + cerebrovascular disease points + dementia points + chronic obstructive pulmonary disease points + hepatic cirrhosis points + cancer points + haemoglobin points. [§]Values higher than maximum or lower than minimum are assigned the listed maximum or minimum values. [¶]Increases were protective in both mortality models. Points are subtracted for higher blood-pressure measurements. [**]Maximum value is equivalent to 21 mmol/L. Score calculated using value in mg/dL.
NA = not applicable to 30-day model.

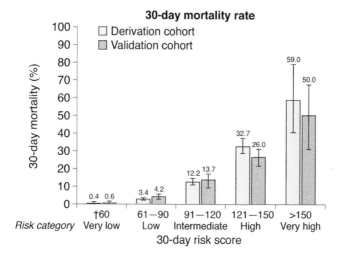

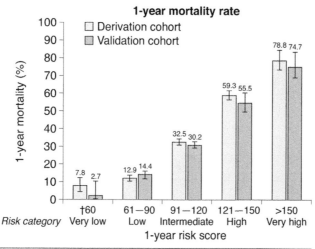

Score categories were assigned according to 30-point increments corresponding to unit SD increments above and below the intermediate range (91—120). Error bars indicate 95% confidence intervals for the mortality rates in each category.

FIGURE 4.1 Mortality rates stratified by 30-day and 1-year risk scores
Source: From the EFFECT study (Lee et al.[25])

Utrecht

A single cohort of patients from seven general hospitals in the Netherlands was studied in a similar way by investigators based in Utrecht.[70] A somewhat different set of parameters emerged, including absence of treatment with beta-blockers (Tables 4.2 and 4.3).

EPICAL

The EPICAL study[60] identified patients with NYHA class III-IV who had been admitted to hospital. The prognostic scoring system that it generated is relatively simple and is summarised in Figure 4.2. It applies primarily to patients with known ischaemia; the paper also gives a slightly different set of criteria that can be applied to those with non-ischaemic cardiomyopathy.

TABLE 4.2 Utrecht: regression coefficient and score of each predictor included in clinical model plus drug treatment at baseline

Predictor	Regression coefficient	Score*
Age (per year)	0.006	0.06
Male sex	0.42	+4
History of diabetes	0.86	+9
History of renal insufficiency	1.65	+17
Ankle oedema	1.03	+10
Weight (per kg)	−0.04	−0.4
Lower systolic or diastolic blood pressure[†]	0.74	+7
Absence of use of beta-blockers	1.30	+13

Notes: *The score per predictor is obtained by multiplying the regression coefficient by 10, and then rounding to nearest integer. †Diastolic blood pressure <70 mmHg or systolic blood pressure <110 mmHg.
Source: With permission of BMJ Publishing Group from Bouvy et al.[70]

TABLE 4.3 Utrecht: distribution of patients according to the risk score derived from model 2

Risk score	Total*	Incidence of mortality (%)[†]	Death[‡]	Survival[‡]
< −15	25	12.0	3	22
≥ −15 and < −5	29	10.3	3	26
≥ −5 and < −1	24	8.3	2	22
≥1 and <7	26	46.2	12	14
≥7 and <11	25	52.0	13	12
≥11	23	78.3	18	5
Total	152		51	101

Notes: Values represent absolute numbers of patients, except for incidence of mortality (%). *Total number of patients per score category. †Observed incidence of mortality per score category. ‡Number of patients who died and survived per score category.
Source: With permission of BMJ Publishing Group from Bouvy et al.[70]

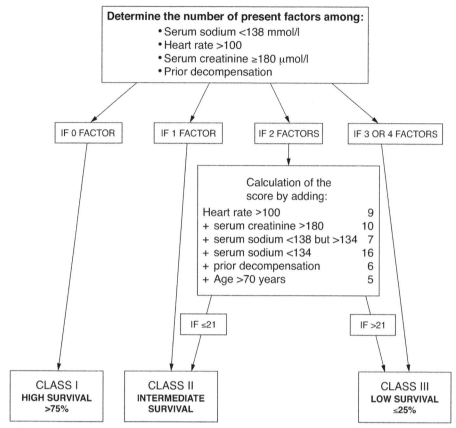

FIGURE 4.2 Epidémiologie de l'Insuffisance Cardiaque Avancée en Lorraine (EPICAL): a clinical scoring system for heart failure due to ischaemic heart disease.
Source: With permission of Elsevier from Alla *et al.*[60]

Chronic Heart Failure Analysis and Registry in Tohoku District (CHART)

CHART is a Japanese prospective observational study of chronic heart failure, which has so far reported only on sudden death as an outcome.[71] The following parameters were found to carry an approximately twofold risk of sudden death:

- non-sustained ventricular tachycardia
- EF <30%
- left ventricular end-diastolic diameter >60 mm
- BNP >200 pg/mL
- diabetes.

Those with three or more of these parameters had a hazard ratio for sudden death of nine, equating to a 3-year risk of about 30%.

HFSS

This score was derived from a cohort of 268 advanced heart failure patients

(NYHA class III or IV). The HFSS consists of seven variables and is used to predict either death or the need for heart transplantation / a ventricular device.[72] It has been validated in at least eight further cohorts,[73] including those on modern treatment such as beta-blockers.[74] However, some of the later validations are less discriminating, and it has been suggested that peak O_2 consumption (a test rarely used unless assessing for heart transplantation) could be replaced by the 6MWT.[73]

Seattle Heart Failure Model

The Seattle Heart Failure Model (SHFM) has been extensively validated.[73] It uses commonly observed clinical characteristics and, unlike the HFSS, has the advantage of not requiring the peak O_2 to calculate a score. Interestingly, renal function was not shown to be an independent predictor in the SHFM. An online calculator is available. BNP was not included in the original model but has been added to a modified version.[75]

MAGGIC

The MAGGIC score was derived from an international database of 30 cohort studies, six of which were clinical trials, and included individual data on 39 372 patients with both reduced and preserved EF, the largest number of patients ever studied in heart failure. Thirteen variables are included in the model, and an online version is available.[76] The authors argue that external validation is not required, as the data were obtained from a large number of patients and studies. However, this score is based on data prior to the widespread use of beta-blockers, aldosterone antagonists or devices (biventricular pacemakers and/or implantable cardiovertor defibrillators). Other criticisms include not considering BNP, large amounts of missing data and the considerable inter-study variability that could not be easily explained.[77] It has been validated in a national heart failure registry.[78]

More detail about validated scores can be found in a systematic review by Alba and colleagues.[73]

Generic tools with heart failure-specific criteria

The challenge of identification of those thought to be in the last 6–12 months of life is not only an issue for heart failure, and generic tools, with varying degrees of validation or none, with disease-specific criteria coupled with clinical prediction are increasingly used in clinical practice. These are summarised well in a systematic review by Maas and colleagues that focuses on the tools available in primary care, such as the Gold Standards Framework (GSF) Prognostic Indicator tool.[79]

A recent study has clearly demonstrated the difficulty in accurately predicting the last year of life in patients with advanced heart failure, with neither the GSF nor the SHFM being useful in a group of community-based ambulatory patients from a clinical database used by heart failure nurse specialists, in a single health authority in Scotland. All patients had NYHA class III or IV symptoms.[12] This study highlights the difficulty in predicting the last year of life in patients with heart failure, even when they are well known to the caregiver and when extensive clinical data are used to predict prognosis. As a predictor of 1-year survival, GSF was poorly specific (specificity of 22%), especially in frail older people. However, it is interesting to note that the GSF Prognostic Indicators identified most patients with palliative care needs, even if they were not those who had less than 1 year to live.

Similarly, another study indicates that the SHFM may be useful to identify patients who may benefit from a specialist palliative care team review rather than to predict death, although its retrospective design limits the conclusions that can be drawn.[80]

SUMMARY

Patients with heart failure have palliative care needs that are not confined to the last year of life.[81] As such, prognostication has limited utility as the primary means to identify heart failure patients who may benefit from a palliative care approach. Instead of continued attempts to predict when patients will die, proposed prospective research should be conducted to identify which patients would benefit from a palliative approach to their care; that is, an assessment of, and attention to, current needs and symptoms and discussions relating to future aims of care.

An estimate of likely survival is useful in that it provides a framework for such discussions about advance care planning, both for medical advance care planning (e.g. device deactivation and determining a ceiling of medical intervention) as well as other issues such as preferred place of care. However, the prognostic uncertainty should be acknowledged, and the estimate of prognosis itself should not necessarily be the gateway through which these conversations may enter.[82] Prognostic research regarding the end of life is possible.[83] Future research regarding prognostication in heart failure is important, apart from any other consideration, because patients would like to know.[84,85]

The two basic questions we need to ask remain: (1) what problems and concerns does this patient have, and (2) is there any reason why I should *not* start thinking about supportive and/or palliative care? These are questions we need to ask about every patient who has had a hospital admission for heart failure.

The risk is that, given the difficulties with prognosis in heart failure, clinicians become paralysed in their ability to do anything other than proceed relentlessly with treatments directed at the heart failure alone rather than seeing the effects on many areas of the patient's life that require help. A problem-oriented approach enables a patient to have access to appropriate services when needed rather than withholding this because 'we're not at that stage yet'. Better prognostic indicators will help in this process, but the fundamental focus should always be on the needs of the individual patient.

REFERENCES

1 Muntwyler J, Abetel G, Gruner C *et al.* One-year mortality among unselected outpatients with heart failure. *Eur Heart J.* 2002; **23**(23): 1861–6.

2 Connors AF, Jr, Dawson NV, Desbiens NA *et al.* A controlled trial to improve care for seriously ill hospitalized patients: the Study to Understand Prognoses and Preferences for Outcomes and Risks of Treatments (SUPPORT). *JAMA.* 1995; **274**(20): 1591–8.

3 Levenson JW, McCarthy EP, Lynn J *et al.* The last six months of life for patients with congestive heart failure. *J Am Geriatr Soc.* 2000; **48**(5 Suppl.):S101–9.

4 Gardner RS. Prognostication. In: McDonagh TA, Gardner RS, Clark AL *et al.*, editors. *Oxford Textbook of Heart Failure.* Oxford: Oxford University Press; 2011. pp. 265–80.

5 Ketchum ES, Levy WC. Establishing prognosis in heart failure: a multimarker approach. *Prog Cardiovasc Dis.* 2011; **54**(2): 86–96.

6 Hemingway H, Riley RD, Altman DG. Ten steps towards improving prognosis research. *BMJ.* 2009; **339**: b4184.

7 Moons KG, Altman DG, Vergouwe Y *et al.* Prognosis and prognostic research: application and impact of prognostic models in clinical practice. *BMJ.* 2009; **338**: b606.

8 Glare P. Predicting and communicating prognosis in palliative care. *BMJ.* 2011; **343**: d5171.

9 Mosterd A, Cost B, Hoes AW *et al.* The prognosis of heart failure in the general population: The Rotterdam Study. *Eur Heart J.* 2001; **22**(15): 1318–27.

10 Senni M, Santilli G, Parrella P *et al.* A novel prognostic index to determine the impact of cardiac conditions and co-morbidities on one-year outcome in patients with heart failure. *Am J Cardiol.* 2006; **98**(8): 1076–82.

11 Levy D, Kenchaiah S, Larson MG *et al.* Long-term trends in the incidence of and survival with heart failure. *N Engl J Med.* 2002; **347**(18): 1397–402.

12 Haga K, Murray S, Reid J *et al.* Identifying community based chronic heart failure patients in the last year of life: a comparison of the Gold Standards Framework Prognostic Indicator Guide and the Seattle Heart Failure Model. *Heart.* 2012; **98**(7): 579–83.

13 Cowie MR, Wood DA, Coats AJ *et al.* Survival of patients with a new diagnosis of heart failure: a population based study. *Heart.* 2000; **83**(5): 505–10.

14 Pocock SJ, McMurray JJ, Dobson J *et al.* Weight loss and mortality risk in patients with chronic heart failure in the Candesartan in Heart failure: Assessment of Reduction in Mortality and morbidity (CHARM) programme. *Eur Heart J.* 2008; **29**(21): 2641–50.

15 Gavazzi A, Berzuini C, Campana C *et al.* Value of right ventricular ejection fraction in predicting short-term prognosis of patients with severe chronic heart failure. *J Heart Lung Transplant.* 1997; **16**(7): 774–85.

16 Pinsky DJ, Sciacca RR, Steinberg JS. QT dispersion as a marker of risk in patients awaiting heart transplantation. *J Am Coll Cardiol.* 1997; **29**(7): 1576–84.

17 Gronda EG, Barbieri P, Frigerio M *et al.* Prognostic indices in heart transplant candidates after the first hospitalization triggered by the need for intravenous pharmacologic circulatory support. *J Heart Lung Transplant.* 1999; **18**(7): 654–63.

18 Abrahamsson P, Dobson J, Granger CB *et al.* Impact of hospitalization for acute coronary events on subsequent mortality in patients with chronic heart failure. *Eur Heart J.* 2009; **30**(3): 338–45.

19 Simon T, Mary-Krause M, Funck-Brentano C et al. Sex differences in the prognosis of congestive heart failure: results from the Cardiac Insufficiency Bisoprolol Study (CIBIS II). Circulation. 2001; 103(3): 375–80.

20 Shahar E, Lee S, Kim J et al. Hospitalized heart failure: rates and long-term mortality. J Card Fail. 2004; 10(5): 374–9.

21 Martínez-Sellés M, Doughty RN, Poppe K et al. Gender and survival in patients with heart failure: interactions with diabetes and aetiology. Results from the MAGGIC individual patient meta-analysis. Eur J Heart Fail. 2012; 14(5): 473–9.

22 Ho KK, Anderson KM, Kannel WB et al. Survival after the onset of congestive heart failure in Framingham Heart Study subjects. Circulation. 1993; 88(1): 107–15.

23 Felker GM, Thompson RE, Hare JM et al. Underlying causes and long-term survival in patients with initially unexplained cardiomyopathy. N Engl J Med. 2000; 342(15): 1077–84.

24 Cubbon RM, Adams B, Rajwani A et al. Diabetes mellitus is associated with adverse prognosis in chronic heart failure of ischaemic and non-ischaemic aetiology. Diab Vasc Dis Res. 2013; 10(4): 330–6.

25 Lee DS, Austin PC, Rouleau JL et al. Predicting mortality among patients hospitalized for heart failure: derivation and validation of a clinical model. JAMA. 2003; 290(19): 2581–7.

26 Rumsfeld JS, Havranek E, Masoudi FA et al. Depressive symptoms are the strongest predictors of short-term declines in health status in patients with heart failure. J Am Coll Cardiol. 2003; 42(10): 1811–17.

27 Mozaffarian D, Nye R, Levy WC. Anemia predicts mortality in severe heart failure: the prospective randomized amlodipine survival evaluation (PRAISE). J Am Coll Cardiol. 2003; 41(11): 1933–9.

28 Gallagher R, Sullivan A, Burke R et al. Mild cognitive impairment, screening, and patient perceptions in heart failure patients. J Card Fail. 2013; 19(9): 641–6.

29 Zuccala G, Onder G, Pedone C et al. Cognitive dysfunction as a major determinant of disability in patients with heart failure: results from a multicentre survey. J Neurol Neurosurg Psychiatry. 2001; 70(1): 109–12.

30 Wang TJ, Larson MG, Levy D et al. Temporal relations of atrial fibrillation and congestive heart failure and their joint influence on mortality: the Framingham Heart Study. Circulation. 2003; 107(23): 2920–5.

31 Crijns HJ, Tjeerdsma G, de Kam PJ et al. Prognostic value of the presence and development of atrial fibrillation in patients with advanced chronic heart failure. Eur Heart J. 2000; 21(15): 1238–45.

32 Kalantar-Zadeh K, Block G, Horwich T et al. Reverse epidemiology of conventional cardiovascular risk factors in patients with chronic heart failure. J Am Coll Cardiol. 2004; 43(8): 1439–44.

33 Gottlieb SS, Abraham W, Butler J et al. The prognostic importance of different definitions of worsening renal function in congestive heart failure. J Card Fail. 2002; 8(3): 136–41.

34 Anker SD, Ponikowski P, Varney S et al. Wasting as independent risk factor for mortality in chronic heart failure. Lancet. 1997; 349(9058): 1050–3.

35 Kenchaiah S, Pocock SJ, Wang D et al. Body mass index and prognosis in patients with chronic heart failure: insights from the Candesartan in Heart failure: Assessment of

Reduction in Mortality and morbidity (CHARM) program. *Circulation.* 2007; **116**(6): 627–36.

36 Gastelurrutia P, Pascual-Figal D, Vazquez R *et al.* Obesity paradox and risk of sudden death in heart failure: results from the MUerte Subita en Insuficiencia Cardiaca (MUSIC) study. *Am Heart J.* 2011; **161**(1): 158–64.

37 O'Connor CM, Whellan DJ, Lee KL *et al.* Efficacy and safety of exercise training in patients with chronic heart failure: HF-ACTION randomized controlled trial. *JAMA.* 2009; **301**(14): 1439–50.

38 Flynn KE, Pina IL, Whellan DJ *et al.* Effects of exercise training on health status in patients with chronic heart failure: HF-ACTION randomized controlled trial. *JAMA.* 2009; **301**(14): 1451–9.

39 Neuberg GW, Miller AB, O'Connor CM *et al.* Diuretic resistance predicts mortality in patients with advanced heart failure. *Am Heart J.* 2002; **144**(1): 31–8.

40 Andreas S, Hagenah G, Möller C *et al.* Cheyne-Stokes respiration and prognosis in congestive heart failure. *Am J Cardiol.* 1996; **78**(11): 1260–4.

41 Lavie CJ, Milani RV, Mehra MR. Peak exercise oxygen pulse and prognosis in chronic heart failure. *Am J Cardiol.* 2004; **93**(5): 588–93.

42 Walsh JT, Charlesworth A, Andrews R *et al.* Relation of daily activity levels in patients with chronic heart failure to long-term prognosis. *Am J Cardiol.* 1997; **79**(10): 1364–9.

43 Bittner V, Weiner DH, Yusuf S *et al.* Prediction of mortality and morbidity with a 6-minute walk test in patients with left ventricular dysfunction. *JAMA.* 1993; **270**(14): 1702–7.

44 Faggiano P, D'Aloia A, Gualeni A *et al.* The 6 minute walking test in chronic heart failure: indications, interpretation and limitations from a review of the literature. *Eur J Heart Fail.* 2004; **6**(6): 687–91.

45 Dunlay SM, Manemann SM, Chamberlain AM *et al.* Activities of daily living and outcomes in heart failure. *Circ Heart Fail.* 2015; **8**(2): 261–7.

46 Nolan J, Batin PD, Andrews R *et al.* Prospective study of heart rate variability and mortality in chronic heart failure: results of the United Kingdom heart failure evaluation and assessment of risk trial (UK-heart). *Circulation.* 1998; **98**(15): 1510–16.

47 La Rovere MT, Pinna GD, Maestri R *et al.* Short-term heart rate variability strongly predicts sudden cardiac death in chronic heart failure patients. *Circulation.* 2003; **107**(4): 565–70.

48 Bilchick KC, Fetics B, Djoukeng R *et al.* Prognostic value of heart rate variability in chronic congestive heart failure (Veterans Affairs' Survival Trial of Antiarrhythmic Therapy in Congestive Heart Failure). *Am J Cardiol.* 2002; **90**(1): 24–8.

49 Tabet JY, Logeart D, Geyer C *et al.* Comparison of the prognostic value of left ventricular filling and peak oxygen uptake in patients with systolic heart failure. *Eur Heart J.* 2000; **21**(22): 1864–71.

50 Florea VG, Henein MY, Cicoira M *et al.* Echocardiographic determinants of mortality in patients >67 years of age with chronic heart failure. *Am J Cardiol.* 2000; **86**(2): 158–61.

51 McMurray JJ, Adamopoulos S, Anker SD *et al.* ESC guidelines for the diagnosis and treatment of acute and chronic heart failure 2012: The Task Force for the Diagnosis

and Treatment of Acute and Chronic Heart Failure 2012 of the European Society of Cardiology. Developed in collaboration with the Heart Failure Association (HFA) of the ESC. *Eur J Heart Fail.* 2012; **14**(8): 803–69.

52 Varadarajan P, Pai RG. Prognosis of congestive heart failure in patients with normal versus reduced ejection fractions: results from a cohort of 2258 hospitalized patients. *J Card Fail.* 2003; **9**(2): 107–12.

53 Anker SD, Doehner W, Rauchhaus M *et al.* Uric acid and survival in chronic heart failure: validation and application in metabolic, functional, and hemodynamic staging. *Circulation.* 2003; **107**(15): 1991–7.

54 Kerzner R, Gage BF, Freedland KE *et al.* Predictors of mortality in younger and older patients with heart failure and preserved or reduced left ventricular ejection fraction. *Am Heart J.* 2003; **146**(2): 286–90.

55 Barnes S, Gott M, Payne S *et al.* Predicting mortality among a general practice-based sample of older people with heart failure. *Chronic Illn.* 2008; **4**(1): 5–12.

56 Gustafsson F, Torp-Pedersen C, Brendorp B *et al.* Long-term survival in patients hospitalized with congestive heart failure: relation to preserved and reduced left ventricular systolic function. *Eur Heart J.* 2003; **24**(9): 863–70.

57 Huynh BC, Rovner A, Rich MW. Long-term survival in elderly patients hospitalized for heart failure: 14-year follow-up from a prospective randomized trial. *Arch Intern Med.* 2006; **166**(17): 1892–8.

58 Kearney MT, Fox KA, Lee AJ *et al.* Predicting death due to progressive heart failure in patients with mild-to-moderate chronic heart failure. *J Am Coll Cardiol.* 2002; **40**(10): 1801–8.

59 Arimoto T, Takeishi Y, Niizeki T *et al.* Cystatin C, a novel measure of renal function, is an independent predictor of cardiac events in patients with heart failure. *J Card Fail.* 2005; **11**(8): 595–601.

60 Alla F, Briancon S, Juilliere Y *et al.* Differential clinical prognostic classifications in dilated and ischemic advanced heart failure: the EPICAL study. *Am Heart J.* 2000; **139**(5): 895–904.

61 Horwich TB, Patel J, MacLellan WR *et al.* Cardiac troponin I is associated with impaired hemodynamics, progressive left ventricular dysfunction, and increased mortality rates in advanced heart failure. *Circulation.* 2003; **108**(7): 833–8.

62 Latini R, Masson S, Anand IS *et al.* Prognostic value of very low plasma concentrations of troponin T in patients with stable chronic heart failure. *Circulation.* 2007; **116**(11): 1242–9.

63 Wang TJ. Significance of circulating troponins in heart failure: if these walls could talk. *Circulation.* 2007; **116**(11): 1217–20.

64 Koglin J, Pehlivanli S, Schwaiblmair M *et al.* Role of brain natriuretic peptide in risk stratification of patients with congestive heart failure. *J Am Coll Cardiol.* 2001; **38**(7): 1934–41.

65 Gardner RS, Ozalp F, Murday AJ *et al.* N-terminal pro-brain natriuretic peptide. A new gold standard in predicting mortality in patients with advanced heart failure. *Eur Heart J.* 2003; **24**(19): 1735–43.

66 Berger R, Huelsman M, Strecker K *et al.* B-type natriuretic peptide predicts sudden death in patients with chronic heart failure. *Circulation.* 2002; **105**(20): 2392–7.

67 Smits JM, Deng MC, Hummel M *et al.* A prognostic model for predicting

waiting-list mortality for a total national cohort of adult heart-transplant candidates. *Transplantation.* 2003; **76**(8): 1185–9.

68   Rector TS, Cohn JN. Assessment of patient outcome with the Minnesota Living with Heart Failure questionnaire: reliability and validity during a randomized, double-blind, placebo-controlled trial of pimobendan. Pimobendan Multicenter Research Group. *Am Heart J.* 1992; **124**(4): 1017–25.

69   Hülsmann M, Berger R, Sturm B *et al.* Prediction of outcome by neurohumoral activation, the six-minute walk test and the Minnesota Living with Heart Failure Questionnaire in an outpatient cohort with congestive heart failure. *Eur Heart J.* 2002; **23**(11): 886–91.

70   Bouvy ML, Heerdink ER, Leufkens HG *et al.* Predicting mortality in patients with heart failure: a pragmatic approach. *Heart.* 2003; **89**(6): 605–9.

71   Watanabe J, Shinozaki T, Shiba N *et al.* Accumulation of risk markers predicts the incidence of sudden death in patients with chronic heart failure. *Eur J Heart Fail.* 2006; **8**(3): 237–42.

72   Aaronson KD, Schwartz JS, Chen TM *et al.* Development and prospective validation of a clinical index to predict survival in ambulatory patients referred for cardiac transplant evaluation. *Circulation.* 1997; **95**(12): 2660–7.

73   Alba AC, Agoritsas T, Jankowski M *et al.* Risk prediction models for mortality in ambulatory patients with heart failure: a systematic review. *Circ Heart Fail.* 2013; **6**(5): 881–9.

74   Koelling TM, Joseph S, Aaronson KD. Heart failure survival score continues to predict clinical outcomes in patients with heart failure receiving beta-blockers. *J Heart Lung Transplant.* 2004; **23**(12): 1414–22.

75   May HT, Horne BD, Levy WC *et al.* Validation of the Seattle Heart Failure Model in a community-based heart failure population and enhancement by adding B-type natriuretic peptide. *Am J Cardiol.* 2007; **100**(4): 697–700.

76   Pocock SJ, Ariti CA, McMurray JJ *et al.* Predicting survival in heart failure: a risk score based on 39 372 patients from 30 studies. *Eur Heart J.* 2013; **34**(19): 1404–13.

77   Braunwald E. Chronic heart failure: a look through the rear view mirror. *Eur Heart J.* 2013; **34**(19): 1391–2.

78   Sartipy U, Dahlström U, Edner M *et al.* Predicting survival in heart failure: validation of the MAGGIC heart failure risk score in 51 043 patients from the Swedish heart failure registry. *Eur J Heart Fail.* 2014; **16**(2): 173–9.

79   Maas EA, Murray SA, Engels Y *et al.* What tools are available to identify patients with palliative care needs in primary care: a systematic literature review and survey of European practice. *BMJ Support Palliat Care.* 2013; **3**(4): 444–51.

80   James T, Offer M, Wilson M. Increasing palliative care consults for heart failure inpatients using the Seattle Heart Failure Model. *J Hosp Palliat Nurs.* 2010; **12**(5): 273–81.

81   Teno JM, Weitzen S, Fennell ML *et al.* Dying trajectory in the last year of life: does cancer trajectory fit other diseases? *J Palliat Med.* 2001; **4**(4): 457–64.

82   Allen LA, Stevenson LW, Grady KL *et al.* Decision making in advanced heart failure: a scientific statement from the American Heart Association. *Circulation.* 2012; **125**(15): 1928–52.

83   Gwilliam B, Keeley V, Todd C *et al.* Development of prognosis in palliative care study

(PiPS) predictor models to improve prognostication in advanced cancer: prospective cohort study. *BMJ.* 2011; **343**: d4920.

84 Harding R, Simms V, Calanzani N *et al.* If you had less than a year to live, would you want to know? A seven-country European population survey of public preferences for disclosure of poor prognosis. *Psychooncology.* 2013; **22**(10):2298–305.

85 Steinhauser KE, Christakis NA, Clipp EC *et al.* Factors considered important at the end of life by patients, family, physicians, and other care providers. *JAMA.* 2000; **284**(19): 2476–82.

CHAPTER 5

Symptom relief for advanced heart failure

WENDY GABRIELLE ANDERSON, STEVE PANTILAT
AND MIRIAM JOHNSON

INTRODUCTION

Patients with advanced heart failure have a high burden of distressing symptoms, which negatively impact their quality of life.[1,2] Over the past 10 years, there has been a *dramatic* increase in research focused specifically on symptom relief in heart failure patients. Some of these studies are small pilot and observational studies, and some larger studies are still underway. Yet this evidence, combined with the wealth of evidence about symptom relief in other illnesses such as cancer,[3] provides a significant developing evidence-based guide to symptom management in advanced heart failure patients.

The first principle is comprehensive symptom assessment, which is part of a global assessment of physical, psychological, social and spiritual needs. This assessment should include a thorough history plus appropriate examination and investigations. The core of the management plan should be explanation and discussion. General and specific treatments should be planned proactively and reviewed regularly. Reversible or underlying causes of symptoms should be treated whenever possible. Issues such as polypharmacy and compliance are important, and the use of self-medication charts and pre-filled weekly drug systems such as dosette boxes may help. For the purposes of this book, we focus on the physical aspects in this chapter and on the psychosocial and spiritual aspects in the next. In practice, of course, there is no such artificial division.

SYMPTOM PREVALENCE AND DISTRESS

Symptom severity forms the basis of the New York Heart Association classification. The symptoms classically associated with heart failure comprise the triad of breathlessness, fatigue and peripheral oedema, which may involve ascites as well as lower limb oedema. In addition, a high frequency of a broad array of symptoms are experienced by patients with advanced heart failure.[1,2,4] The most prevalent symptoms, reported by more than half of patients, include breathlessness, lack of energy, pain, drowsiness and dry mouth (*see* Table 5.1). Symptoms are more prevalent in patients with more advanced disease. On average, each patient experiences 9–12 symptoms, and half of patients report high symptom-related distress. Higher numbers of symptoms and higher levels of symptom distress are both associated with lower quality of life and the presence of depression and psychological distress.

TABLE 5.1 Common symptoms in heart failure patients

Symptom	Prevalence (%)[1,2,4]
Lack of energy	62–70
Breathlessness	56–65
Feeling drowsy	52
Dry mouth	50–73
Numbness/Tingling in hands and feet	48–55
Difficulty sleeping	44–7
Worrying	44–50
Cough	40–5
Feeling sad	38–43
Pain	38–52
Change in taste	25–50
Weight loss	15–52

OPTIMISATION OF MEDICAL MANAGEMENT

The cornerstone of symptom management for heart failure is ensuring that patients are taking the optimum tolerated medical treatment (*see* Chapter 3, 'Optimal therapy for heart failure'). Even in the dying phase (*see* Chapter 8, 'Care of the patient dying from heart failure'), patients are likely to need a loop diuretic and perhaps nitrates (furosemide given subcutaneously and nitrates transdermally when the intravenous route becomes difficult or inappropriate) to control breathlessness, oedema and angina, in addition to opioids and benzodiazepines.

There is clear evidence that many patients with heart failure are suboptimally managed in terms of the evidence-based therapies such as angiotensin-converting enzyme inhibitors, beta-blockers and spironolactone.[5] The situation is exacerbated by the common problems of each admission being under the care of a different physician, with seemingly no one grasping an overview of the clinical progression, and of poor monitoring that fails to sustain improvements made. Fluid status (sometimes helped by defining the 'dry weight' of a person) and renal function require monitoring, and diuretics often require frequent adjustment. Any individual's management plan needs to consider not only cognition, compliance and polypharmacy issues but also the challenges presented by co-morbidities. Optimal medical management for most heart failure patients therefore also includes management of co-morbidities such as peripheral vascular disease, chronic obstructive pulmonary disease (COPD), diabetes, arthritis, renal failure and depression.[6] Clearly, professionals need to be not only aware of each other but also able to work together.

INTEGRATED CARE DELIVERY SYSTEMS

The need for palliative care in heart failure has been widely recognised,[7,8] and there is growing evidence that patients with heart failure who receive palliative care have lower symptom distress and other improvements in outcomes.[9-11] Yet we must be cautious to create care models that integrate palliative care within systems that address all patients' care needs (*see* Chapter 10, 'Palliative care services for patients with heart failure'). Patients and their caregivers identify needs for symptoms management and other palliative care needs.[12] Yet many patients may find it difficult to attend palliative care clinics in addition to their primary care and specialty appointments,[9] and patients and their caregivers usually prefer that this care be coordinated by a provider who knows them well and also understands their heart failure.[12]

Thus, effective care models will integrate a broad range of disciplines and specialties including cardiology, primary care, palliative care, rehabilitation, nursing, social work, psychiatry and psychology, and spiritual care.[6,13] Further, this integrated care must be delivered across a range of settings, including the outpatient clinic, the hospital, long-term care and home settings.[14,15] In some countries, such as the USA, this will require the design of new care models, as palliative care is well developed in hospital consultation and hospice programmes but less well developed in the outpatient setting.[16] Though palliative care interventions may decrease the frequency of hospital care and help patients die at home if they want to,[11] services need to be designed so that patients can have both the best heart failure management and the best palliative care management – including advanced therapies – without having to choose between the two. This will require cardiology clinicians to be educated in palliative care, and home care and palliative care clinicians to be educated in the principles of heart failure management.[17]

THERAPEUTIC OPTIONS FOR COMMON SYMPTOMS

Table 5.2 briefly lists practical tips for symptom control in heart failure.

TABLE 5.2 Tips for symptom control in heart failure

Symptom	Simple symptom control options
Breathlessness	<ul><li>Optimally treat heart failure and co-morbid diseases, including anxiety</li><li>Exercise rehabilitation</li><li>Opioids:<ul><li>oral morphine 2.5–5.0 mg 4 hourly and titrate</li><li>manage common opioid side effects</li><li>seek advice if renal function poor or opioid toxicity</li></ul></li></ul>
Fatigue	<ul><li>Search for reversible factors</li><li>Consider treatment of anaemia</li><li>Appropriate exercise</li><li>Avoid steroids and progestogens</li></ul>
Pain	<ul><li>Avoid NSAIDs and tricyclic antidepressants</li><li>Use the WHO analgesic ladder:[18] follow Step 1, then 2, then 3 (all drugs oral):<ul><li>Step 1: paracetamol 1 g qds. Caplets or tablets</li><li>Step 2: paracetamol 500 mg + codeine 30 mg, two tablets qds *or* tramadol 50–100 mg qds ± regular paracetamol</li><li>Step 3: morphine 5–10 mg 4 hourly and prn. Titrate every 48 hours if pain not controlled</li></ul></li></ul>Manage common opioid side effects. Seek advice if renal function poor, opioid toxicity or good pain control not achieved
Nausea and vomiting	<ul><li>Search for reversible factors</li><li>Oral metoclopramide 10 mg tds or haloperidol 1.5–3.0 mg od</li><li>Avoid cyclizine</li></ul>
Constipation	<ul><li>Laxative:<ul><li>first-line: stimulant (senna); provide routinely to all patients taking opioids</li><li>second-line: surfactant (lactulose, polyethylene glycol)</li></ul></li></ul>
Dry mouth	<ul><li>Avoid acids</li><li>Mucin-based saliva substitutes, sugar-free chewing gum</li></ul>
Skin problems	<ul><li>Aqueous cream as soap substitute and moisturiser</li><li>2% menthol in aqueous cream for itch</li></ul>
Depression	<ul><li>Have a low index of suspicion for depression</li><li>Consider non-drug approaches</li><li>Avoid tricyclic antidepressants and drugs with many potential drug interactions (e.g. fluoxetine)</li><li>Sertraline 50 mg od, citalopram 10–20 mg od, mirtazapine 15–30 mg od</li></ul>

NSAIDs = non-steroidal anti-inflammatory drugs; od = once daily; prn = as needed; qds = four times daily; tds = three times daily; WHO = World Health Organization.

BREATHLESSNESS

Breathlessness is one of the most serious concerns, from the terrifying experience of paroxysmal nocturnal dyspnoea to the debilitating breathlessness on exertion. It is closely allied to muscle weakness and fatigue, and even patients who are at dry weight may experience limiting breathlessness.

Assessment

Potentially reversible factors should be looked for and treated. For example, persistent pleural effusion despite diuretics may need drainage, and chest infections should be treated with antibiotics. A chest X-ray may be useful. Most patients with heart failure have a history of smoking and may well have coexistent obstructive airway disease or may even develop bronchogenic carcinoma. It is important to look for and manage associated anxiety, as panic may be a significant exacerbating factor. Ascites and an engorged liver can restrict diaphragmatic movement and inspiration.

General measures

There is increasing evidence for the effectiveness of non-pharmacological intervention, including mindfulness-based interventions and exercise training, to improve the management of breathlessness.[19,20] Mindfulness programmes can also improve anxiety and depression,[21] and exercise training programmes decrease hospitalisations and improve quality of life.[22] Programmes are increasingly available in hospitals, hospices and patients' homes.[22] The focus of non-pharmacological evaluation and intervention should be broad, including understanding what breathlessness means for the individual, breathing exercises to train for more effective respiration for those with dysfunctional breathing patterns, assisting adaptation to better ways of coping with associated fear and panic through relaxation techniques, pacing of activities and even the simple use of a fan. Restrictive undergarments are still discovered on occasion, particularly in older people; persuading the patient to discard these may help. The potential benefit from a thorough social and practical needs review, with referral on to therapy, welfare and social services, as appropriate, cannot be overstated and is discussed more fully in Chapter 6, 'Supportive care: psychological, social and spiritual aspects'.

Specific measures
Opioids

Morphine has been used empirically for many years to relieve symptoms in acute left ventricular failure or myocardial ischaemia. Opioids are postulated to improve breathlessness through reduction in chemoreceptor hypersensitivity and subsequent improvement in the abnormal ventilatory patterns found in heart failure.[23] Haemodynamic effects are not thought to be important.[24] Physicians may be less comfortable with the use of opioids for dyspnoea than for pain, especially in patients who are not actively dying,[25] although patients with heart failure seem to be less concerned if advised to take opioids by a trusted clinician.[26]

A systematic review of studies of opioids for refractory breathlessness found evidence to support the use of oral or parenteral, but not nebulised, opioids based on small studies.[27] These studies were conducted in mixed populations of patients with serious illness, including primarily COPD, as well as cancer and heart failure.[27] A subsequent adequately powered crossover trial confirmed benefit in a mixed population.[28] Low doses (10–30 mg per day) of sustained-release morphine are well tolerated and effective for the relief of dyspnoea in many patients.[28,29] The main side effect is constipation. A dose-titration and pharmacovigilance study found a response rate of 62%, with over 90% of responders achieving benefit with a daily dose of 20 mg.[29] Though many patients responded to sustained-release morphine within 24 hours, continued improvement was observed for up to 7 days, indicating that doses should not be titrated more frequently than once per week when treating chronic dyspnoea.[30] A retrospective analysis of pooled datasets from four clinical trials of opioids for chronic refractory breathlessness, with equal numbers of patients with COPD and heart failure, found that patients with higher baseline breathlessness intensity and younger age were more likely to respond, and that the cause of the breathlessness did *not* predict response.[31]

Two trials of opioids for the relief of dyspnoea have focused on heart failure patients.[32,33] A controlled double-blind crossover trial of 35 patients with New York Heart Association class III–IV chronic heart failure found no effect of 4 days of oral morphine (5 mg four times per day) or oxycodone (2.5 mg four times per day) on breathlessness.[33] Both opioids were well tolerated and did not cause any deterioration in patients' clinical conditions. However, a 3-month open-label extension of this study, in which 33 of the original participants were followed for 3 months and allowed to continue open-label opioids if they wished, found a significant improvement in breathlessness in the 13 patients who chose to continue opioids, compared with the 20 who did not.[32] Opioids were also well tolerated in this study, and patients in the opioid group also had an improvement in global assessment of change in their dyspnoea, as well as their physical quality of life.

A 3-month randomised controlled trial of sustained-release morphine for refractory breathlessness in heart failure patients will begin in 2015 and will include a 1-year open-label follow-up.[34] The Cochrane systematic review evaluating the effectiveness of opioids for treating dyspnoea in patients with chronic heart failure is currently being updated.[35]

As breathlessness is integrally related to exertion and skeletal muscle condition, the role of opioids for the use of exertion-related breathlessness shows potential.[36]

Benzodiazepines

The use of benzodiazepines, prescribed both on a scheduled and as-needed basis, is common in palliative care. A 2010 systematic review addressed the effectiveness of benzodiazepines for the relief of breathlessness in advanced malignant and non-malignant diseases.[37] Identified studies included patients with cancer and COPD. A meta-analysis found no beneficial effect of benzodiazepines for the relief of breathlessness, though the authors noted a non-significant trend towards a beneficial effect but with a small effect size. Thus, the authors recommend using a benzodiazepine as a second- or third-line agent for breathlessness.

Certainly, caution should be used in prescribing benzodiazepines in patients with heart failure, given the potentially serious problems of memory loss, falls, tolerance and addiction with chronic use, particularly in frail older people. Patients with significant anxiety, depression or panic attacks (when breathlessness spirals out of control) should first be treated with the specific breathing control and relaxation techniques of pulmonary rehabilitation, and, if drug treatment is needed, anxiolytics – such as selective serotonin reuptake inhibitor antidepressants (e.g. citalopram) – which are known to be safe in heart failure, can be used. Results from an ongoing study of sertraline for a mixed population with refractory breathlessness will be interesting.[38] In appropriate cases, judicious use of an intermediate-acting benzodiazepine, such as lorazepam or lormetazepam, to gain control of panic in addition to the just mentioned may be useful. Lorazepam tablets can, in fact, be quickly absorbed sublingually.

Oxygen

Oxygen therapy is considered part of the first-line management of acute left heart failure in addition to diuretics and opioids. However, for heart failure patients, recommendations do not routinely include oxygen therapy. Arterial desaturation and hypoxia on exercise are not common in patients with compensated heart failure. Lung disease is common in many patients with heart failure, and these patients may gain some symptomatic benefit from oxygen therapy because of that. A body of literature has examined the impact of oxygen on breathlessness in patients with advanced illness who are not hypoxaemic or mildly hypoxaemic. These studies, which have focused mostly on patients with cancer and COPD,[39-42] have concluded that oxygen does not improve breathlessness in patients with cancer who are not hypoxaemic, although there may be some benefit for people with COPD.[41] Studies specifically looking at the benefits of oxygen on the sensation of breathlessness in severe heart failure are ongoing. The practicalities of providing ambulatory oxygen should be remembered in considering cost–benefit balance in addition to the psychological dependence that can occur for such patients – some patients become psychologically dependent on oxygen therapy, even when it is of doubtful benefit, creating panic if there is a problem with supply. Thus, decisions need to be made on an individual patient basis, taking into account all factors.[43]

FATIGUE

Fatigue is the other major complaint of patients with chronic heart failure and can be difficult to improve. Again, the principle of a full assessment, looking for reversible factors, is important. Table 5.3 lists the common ones.

TABLE 5.3 Fatigue in heart failure: common potentially reversible factors

Diuretics	Over-diuresis
	Hypokalaemia
Beta-blockers	Tiredness
Sleep disorders	Orthopnoea, paroxysmal dyspnoea, sleep apnoea and nocturnal hypoventilation
Depression	
Anaemia	
Exercise deconditioning	

Timing and amount of diuretics can impinge on quality of sleep. This, and sleep disorders due to other reasons, can impact on daytime wakefulness.

Sleep apnoea and nocturnal hypoventilation are important to diagnose, as some patients gain benefit from non-invasive ventilation at night. Patients with heart failure may not complain of classic symptoms, such as morning headache and daytime somnolence; evaluation with overnight polysomnography should be prompted by obesity and refractory hypertension in men; women may have unexplained pulmonary hypertension or tricuspid regurgitation.[44] Treatment with continuous positive airway pressure can improve quality of life for patients with heart failure and obstructive sleep apnoea.[44] A trial in patients with central sleep apnoea and heart failure found that although continuous positive airway pressure did not affect survival, it did increase walking distance, nocturnal oxygenation and ejection fraction.[45]

It has become increasingly accepted that muscle bulk and function play a very important role in the symptoms of heart failure and that exercise is beneficial. Exercise training improves fatigue as well as breathlessness and quality of life for patients with heart failure.[20,22,46] Patients may need reassurance and encouragement, as they may be very nervous of physical exercise, worried it may cause further cardiac events. Prioritisation and pacing of activities can be very helpful; many patients need assistance to adjust to their limitations, so that they become less frustrating. Without such help, heart failure patients can become stuck in a cycle of physical inactivity and progressive limitation, which can contribute to depression and social isolation. A systematic review examined 11 small randomised controlled trials of neuromuscular electrical stimulation in patients with advanced illness including chronic heart failure. Neuromuscular electrical stimulation improved both muscle strength as well as walk tests, indicating that it may help with function and the ability to participate in exercise programmes.[47]

Many patients with heart failure have anaemia as well as iron deficiency. Randomised controlled trials examined intravenous iron supplementation in patients with heart failure and iron deficiency, regardless of whether they had anaemia.[48,49] The intravenous iron treatment improved quality of life and walking distance, decreased hospitalisations and was not associated with significant adverse events. A further randomised controlled trial found that in patients with systolic failure who have mild-to-moderate anaemia of unknown aetiology and are iron-replete, correction of anaemia with the erythropoietin-stimulating agent darbepoetin alfa did not reduce the rate of death or hospitalisation but did increase the risk of thromboembolic events.[50] Thus, the risk of routine correction of mild-to-moderate anaemia of chronic disease with transfusions or erythropoietin-stimulating agents likely outweighs any benefits.

PAIN

Pain is an often under-recognised symptom in heart failure that can be prevalent, severe and prolonged. Pain can be cardiac (angina pectoris) and non-cardiac (musculoskeletal pain, dyspepsia, gout, peripheral vascular disease, from oedematous legs or tense ascites). The assessment and management of pain need to follow the basic principles laid out at the beginning of this chapter.

Non-cardiac pain

The management of chronic pain, both in malignant and non-malignant disease, requires the regular administration of analgesics, titrated up to achieve effective pain control. A combination of drugs with different actions is often required. The World Health Organization (WHO) three-step analgesic ladder provides an excellent framework with which to start[51] (*see* Box 5.1).

BOX 5.1 World Health Organization analgesic ladder

Step 1 Mild pain	Non-opioid ± adjuvant	E.g. paracetamol 1 g qds
Step 2 Moderate pain	Mild opioid + non-opioid ± adjuvant	E.g. co-codamol 30/500 two tablets qds
Step 3 Severe pain	Strong opioid ± adjuvant	E.g. morphine given regularly, dose titrated to individual patient need

qds = four times daily.

Step 1 is paracetamol, which should be given regularly at a dose of 1 g four times a day. Step 2 is to add or substitute a weak opioid, such as codeine, dihydrocodeine or tramadol. Fixed-combination tablets of weak opioid and paracetamol can be useful aids to acceptability and compliance, but those with a sub-therapeutic dose of opioid should be avoided – that is, use paracetamol 500 mg plus codeine 30 mg, two tablets four times a day. If this is ineffective, do not swap to another weak opioid but move up to the next step.

Step 3 is for strong opioids. Sometimes paracetamol will still have an additive effect on pain and can be continued. Weak opioids should be stopped when strong opioids are started. Oral morphine remains the strong opioid of choice – although, as it is renally excreted, additional care must be taken in the presence of renal dysfunction. Morphine can be taken as an immediate-release tablet or liquid regularly four hourly or as a modified-release preparation. Both 12-hourly and 24-hourly preparations are available. Immediate-release morphine is often used initially to titrate to the dose required, then the patient is transferred on to a modified-release preparation. Once stable, immediate-release morphine must still be prescribed for any breakthrough pain, the dose being one-sixth of the total 24-hour dose. However, a randomised controlled trial comparing titration with sustained-release and immediate-release morphine showed that time to adequate relief was quicker in the sustained-release group.[52] Patients who have been on the maximum dose of a weak opioid – such as codeine 60 mg four times a day – but are still in pain will usually require at least oral morphine 10 mg four hourly on transfer to step 3. A lower dose may be used if the patient, carer or clinician is not confident in the use of morphine, but up-titration performed quickly if necessary.

Common side effects of opioids (weak and strong) should be anticipated and treated. Most patients get constipated and need regular laxatives. Initial nausea occurs in about a third of patients, and prompt access to an anti-emetic such as metoclopramide should be provided. Drowsiness should wear off after 2–3 days but will often recur at each up-titration. Affected patients should be counselled not to drive during the first week of therapy and when the dose is further increased, if thus affected, but there are no specific driving restrictions in patients who are not drowsy on stable morphine. The use of alternative strong opioids is beyond the scope of this text. Their use will usually require advice from clinicians familiar with them, such as those from specialist palliative care.

Non-aspirin, non-steroidal anti-inflammatory drugs (NSAIDs) are contraindicated in heart failure patients because of their fluid-retaining side effects. By expanding the intravascular volume, NSAIDs also blunt the response to diuretics. One study showed a doubling of the risk of hospital admission for worsening heart failure in previously stable patients who were started on a NSAID.[53] There were no differences between NSAIDs, and no dose response was observed. The risk of admission was highest within the first few days of initiation, and usually happened within 30 days. The risk of gastrointestinal bleeding is also greater in patients with significant co-morbidity such as heart failure. Many of these patients also have renal dysfunction or are on a combination of a loop diuretic and angiotensin-converting enzyme inhibitor – adding a NSAID to this cocktail is potentially nephrotoxic, particularly in older people. Therefore, it is recommended that *all* NSAIDs be avoided in heart failure patients. Restricting the use of NSAIDs can make the management of arthritis difficult but not impossible, as application of the WHO analgesic ladder is appropriate and applicable. The treatment of gout can be managed with colchicine, although almost all patients develop diarrhoea within 48 hours of the dose required. This can be disastrous in patients with poor mobility and may result in the humiliation of faecal incontinence.

Some pains do not respond fully to conventional analgesics. Neuropathic pain is the classic example, but, in practice, this is also true of the pain of tender, sore legs in heart failure. Adjuvant analgesics are usually required. Tricyclic antidepressants have a better profile of effectiveness and side effects than anticonvulsants, but tricyclics are relatively contraindicated in heart failure because of their anticholinergic activity. Thus, an anticonvulsant such as gabapentin is safest in heart failure. Again, its use will usually require advice from clinicians familiar with it, such as those from specialist palliative care.

Cardiac pain

The pain from angina pectoris is usually controlled with anti-anginal medication, but there are patients for who this remains a severe and limiting problem despite optimal treatment. Intravenous diamorphine is well accepted in the relief of acute ischaemic cardiac pain. However, although morphine is effective in chronic pain, there is a reluctance to use it, partly again because of a paucity of literature confirming efficacy and safety. A small prospective study of 12 patients attending a regional refractory angina clinic demonstrated successful titration of sustained-release preparations of morphine or oxycodone (for those with unacceptable drowsiness or pruritus).[54] These patients had failed to respond to psychological therapies, transcutaneous nerve stimulation, and temporary sympathetic blockade. Patients were followed up for 12 weeks. Only two patients were unable to tolerate opioids because of sedation and nausea. Frequency of angina and total pain burden was reduced with a corresponding increase in exercise capacity, general health and vitality. Significantly, an improvement was also seen in depression score and social functioning, highlighting the impact of chronic physical symptoms. Opioids were well tolerated and low risk in these patients in this setting.

Transcutaneous nerve stimulation has also been used with some success in intractable angina but has not become commonplace.[55] Studies are difficult to conduct (it is hard to blind treatment) and the placebo effect is high. However, reports suggest it improves pain, diminishes ST-segment changes and affects regional coronary blood flow.

Spinal-cord stimulation may improve symptoms of angina and improve quality of life, as well as reduce hospitalisations.[56] A pilot randomised controlled trial of spinal-cord stimulation in refractory angina is underway.[57] Patient selection is of paramount importance, and the procedure (which usually requires general anaesthesia) carries risks of infection and haematoma formation. Many such patients are anticoagulated, which adds to the difficulty.

CONSTIPATION

Constipation is common due to reduced mobility, restricted fluid and food intake, diuresis and opioids. Many patients are fluid restricted, which can create problems with ispaghula husk. Patients prescribed opioids should routinely be prescribed a stimulant laxative such as senna. Though docusate has been widely prescribed in palliative care, research indicates that it may have side effects, including nausea, increase pill burden and not add benefit compared with senna alone.[58] For patients who receive significant benefit from opioids but have intractable constipation, methylnaltrexone may be considered;[59,60] the cost and the requirement that this medication be given by injection limit its use. For patients with intractable constipation, attention should also be paid to reducing anticholinergic medications, which are, in any case, relatively contraindicated in heart failure due to their pro-arrhythmic potential.[61]

ANOREXIA / CACHEXIA, NAUSEA, DRY MOUTH

Anorexia is a troublesome issue. A commonsense approach, again looking for reversible problems – such as oral candida, untreated nausea or constipation, and ill-fitting teeth due to weight loss – is important. Sometimes patients are not eating enough because they do not have the energy to prepare themselves a meal, and the practical step of getting help in this regard may be all that is needed. Small meals attractively presented and the avoidance of cooking smells, if possible, are often helpful, as is altering practice to grazing on smaller snacks during the day. Improved management of symptoms, including breathlessness, pain and depression, may help as well.

Sometimes, the issue of food intake can cause distressing conflict between carers and the patient. As meal times are inherently part of our whole family / social structure, tensions can arise and patients feel under pressure to eat. A common approach of eating for enjoyment, little and often may take the pressure off the patient. However, this will entail an honest discussion regarding the stage of disease, which many professionals find difficult. Nevertheless, before this supervenes, it is important to pay attention to diet, as there is evidence that some patients with clinically stable heart failure are in negative calorie balance.[62] In this situation, advice from a dietician may be beneficial. Patients may also benefit from amino acid supplementation.[63] Weight loss that is clearly not due to diuresis is a poor sign and may indicate that the anorexia is part of the cachexia syndrome of advanced heart failure. The syndrome is caused by inflammatory cytokines and leads to a catabolic/anabolic imbalance.[64] There is little evidence to suggest that increasing calorie intake *at this advanced stage* is likely to have benefit.

Patients can be nauseated due to drug side effects (aspirin, spironolactone, digoxin toxicity, opioids), gut-wall or liver congestion, or renal failure. A prokinetic anti-emetic such as metoclopramide (10 mg three times daily) may help both situations and is probably more reliably absorbed from the gut than domperidone. Domperidone does come in suppository form, which is occasionally useful if a patient is vomiting, wishes to stay at home and does not want a syringe driver for subcutaneous administration. A good alternative to metoclopramide would be low-dose haloperidol (0.5–3.0 mg), which can be used once daily at night. If possible, anti-emetics with a strong anticholinergic action should be avoided (such as cyclizine or hyoscine) because of potential cardiac toxicity and exacerbation of constipation.

A dry mouth (xerostomia) may be due to drugs, particularly diuretics, analgesics and anti-emetics. Mucin-based saliva substitutes and using sugar-free chewing gum as a saliva stimulant may be helpful. Avoid acids in dentate patients, either in artificial saliva, vitamin C or fruit juices, since they cause demineralisation of teeth and other oral problems. Look for and treat oral candida.

SKIN CARE (CELLULITIS, DRY/ITCHY SKIN, OEDEMA)

Skin care is an overlooked problem. Chronic peripheral oedema can result in dry, thinned, friable skin at risk of cellulitis. Co-morbidities such as diabetes or peripheral vascular disease may also complicate the picture by adding poor peripheral circulation. In general, the patient's skin may become dry and itchy. Simple measures such as regular application of aqueous cream or similar moisturiser can help. The addition of menthol, as a cooling agent, to the cream can give further benefit.

Sometimes itch may be present because of concomitant renal failure. A large number of small studies, often case series, have been conducted to assess the effectiveness of various medications on pruritus in palliative care patients.[65] While there is no high-quality evidence for any medication, a few medications may be trialled: paroxetine, the selective serotonin reuptake inhibitor for general itching of undetermined origin; gabapentin or the kappa-opioid receptor agonist nalfurafine for chronic kidney disease patients, rifampicin and flumecinol for cholestatic pruritus; and the opioid antagonist naltrexone for uraemic or cholestatic pruritus. Naltrexone may not be feasible in patients who are taking opioids, because it will lessen their efficacy.

SUMMARY

Patients with advanced heart failure have a high burden of distressing symptoms, which negatively affect their quality of life. Common physical symptoms are breathlessness, fatigue and pain. The cornerstone of symptom management for heart failure is ensuring optimum medical treatment. There is a growing evidence base to guide treatment of specific symptoms. Integrated care delivery systems including a broad range of disciplines and specialties are essential to addressing symptom needs for patients with heart failure across the continuum of care.

REFERENCES

1 Bekelman DB, Havranek EP, Becker DM *et al*. Symptoms, depression, and quality of life in patients with heart failure. *J Card Fail*. 2007; 13(8): 643–8.
2 Blinderman CD, Homel P, Billings JA *et al*. Symptom distress and quality of life in

patients with advanced congestive heart failure. *J Pain Symptom Manage.* 2008; **35**(6): 594–603.

3 Hanks G, Cherny NI, Christakis NA *et al.*, editors. *Oxford Textbook of Palliative Medicine.* 4th ed. Oxford: Oxford University Press; 2010.

4 Wilson J, McMillan S. Symptoms experienced by heart failure patients in hospice care. *J Hosp Palliat Nurs.* 2013; **15**(1): 13–21.

5 Fonarow GC. How well are chronic heart failure patients being managed? *Rev Cardiovasc Med.* 2006; 7 Suppl. 1:S3–11.

6 Smith SM, Soubhi H, Fortin M *et al.* Interventions for improving outcomes in patients with multimorbidity in primary care and community settings. *Cochrane Database Syst Rev.* 2012; **4**: CD006560.

7 Goodlin SJ,Hauptman PJ, Arnold R *et al.* Consensus statement: palliative and supportive care in advanced heart failure. *J Card Fail.* 2004; **10**(3): 200–9.

8 Pantilat SZ,Steimle AE. Palliative care for patients with heart failure. *JAMA.* 2004; **291**(20): 2476–82.

9 Evangelista LS, Liao S, Motie M *et al.* On-going palliative care enhances perceived control and patient activation and reduces symptom distress in patients with symptomatic heart failure: a pilot study. *Eur J Cardiovasc Nurs.* 2014; **13**(2): 116–23.

10 Schwarz ER, Baraghoush A, Morrissey RP *et al.* Pilot study of palliative care consultation in patients with advanced heart failure referred for cardiac transplantation. *J Palliat Med.* 2012; **15**(1): 12–15.

11 Pattenden JF, Mason AR, Lewin RJ. Collaborative palliative care for advanced heart failure: outcomes and costs from the 'Better Together' pilot study. *BMJ Support Palliat Care.* 2013; **3**(1): 69–76.

12 Bekelman DB, Nowels CT, Retrum JH *et al.* Giving voice to patients' and family caregivers' needs in chronic heart failure: implications for palliative care programs. *J Palliat Med.* 2011; **14**(12): 1317–24.

13 Bekelman DB, Hooker S, Nowels CT *et al.* Feasibility and acceptability of a collaborative care intervention to improve symptoms and quality of life in chronic heart failure: mixed methods pilot trial. *J Palliat Med.* 2014; **17**(2): 145–51.

14 Takeda A, Taylor SJ, Taylor RS *et al.* Clinical service organisation for heart failure. *Cochrane Database Syst Rev.* 2012; **9**: CD002752.

15 Bekelman DB, Plomondon ME, Sullivan MD *et al.* Patient-centered disease management (PCDM) for heart failure: study protocol for a randomised controlled trial. *BMC Cardiovasc Disord.* 2013; **13**: 49.

16 Morrison RS. Models of palliative care delivery in the United States. *Curr Opin Support Palliat Care.* 2013; **7**(2): 201–6.

17 Delaney C, Apostolidis B, Lachapelle L *et al.* Home care nurses' knowledge of evidence-based education topics for management of heart failure. *Heart Lung.* 2011; **40**(4): 285–92.

18 WHO. *Cancer Pain Relief; with a guide to opioid availability.* 2nd ed. Geneva; 1996.

19 Johnson MJ, Oxberry SG. The management of dyspnoea in chronic heart failure. *Curr Opin Support Palliat Care.* 2010; **4**(2): 63–8.

20 McConnell TR, Mandak JS, Sykes JS *et al.* Exercise training for heart failure patients improves respiratory muscle endurance, exercise tolerance, breathlessness, and quality of life. *J Cardiopulm Rehabil.* 2003; **23**(1): 10–16.

21 Sullivan MJ, Wood L, Terry J *et al.* The Support, Education, and Research in Chronic Heart Failure Study (SEARCH): a mindfulness-based psychoeducational intervention improves depression and clinical symptoms in patients with chronic heart failure. *Am Heart J.* 2009; **157**(1): 84–90.

22 Taylor RS, Sagar VA, Davies EJ *et al.* Exercise-based rehabilitation for heart failure. *Cochrane Database Syst Rev.* 2014; 4: CD003331.

23 Chua TP, Harrington D, Ponikowski P *et al.* Effects of dihydrocodeine on chemosensitivity and exercise tolerance in patients with chronic heart failure. *J Am Coll Cardiol.* 1997; **29**(1): 147–52.

24 Timmis AD, Rothman MT, Henderson MA *et al.* Haemodynamic effects of intravenous morphine in patients with acute myocardial infarction complicated by severe left ventricular failure. *Br Med J.* 1980; **280**(6219): 980–2.

25 Hadjiphilippou S, Odogwu SE, Dand P. Doctors' attitudes towards prescribing opioids for refractory dyspnoea: a single-centred study. *BMJ Support Palliat Care.* Epub ahead of print: 6 March 2014.

26 Oxberry SG, Jones L, Clark AL *et al.* Attitudes to morphine in chronic heart failure patients. *Postgrad Med J.* 2012; **88**(1043): 515–21.

27 Jennings AL, Davies AN, Higgins JP *et al.* A systematic review of the use of opioids in the management of dyspnoea. *Thorax.* 2002; **57**(11): 939–44.

28 Abernethy AP, Currow DC, Frith P *et al.* Randomised, double blind, placebo controlled crossover trial of sustained release morphine for the management of refractory dyspnoea. *BMJ.* 2003; **327**(7414): 523–8.

29 Currow DC, McDonald C, Oaten S *et al.* Once-daily opioids for chronic dyspnea: a dose increment and pharmacovigilance study. *J Pain Symptom Manage.* 2011; **42**(3): 388–99.

30 Currow DC, Quinn S, Greene A *et al.* The longitudinal pattern of response when morphine is used to treat chronic refractory dyspnea. *J Palliat Med.* 2013; **16**(8): 881–6.

31 Johnson MJ, Bland JM, Oxberry SG *et al.* Opioids for chronic refractory breathlessness: patient predictors of beneficial response. *Eur Respir J.* 2013; **42**(3): 758–66.

32 Oxberry SG, Bland JM, Clark AL *et al.* Repeat dose opioids may be effective for breathlessness in chronic heart failure if given for long enough. *J Palliat Med.* 2013; **16**(3): 250–5.

33 Oxberry SG, Torgerson DJ, Bland JM *et al.* Short-term opioids for breathlessness in stable chronic heart failure: a randomized controlled trial. *Eur J Heart Fail.* 2011; **13**(9): 1006–12.

34 Hull and East Yorkshire Hospitals NHS Trust (UK). Morphine for the relief of breathlessness in chronic heart failure (CHF) [clinical trial]. ISRCTN identifier: 41349358. In: ISRCTN Registry [website]. London: BioMed Central; 2014 [updated 19 May 2014]. Available at: www.isrctn.com/ISRCTN41349358 (accessed 8 May 2015).

35 Shearer FA, Struthers AD, Harbour RT. Opioids for treating dyspnoea in patients with chronic heart failure. *Cochrane Database Syst Rev.* 2014; (2): CD010991.

36 Johnson MJ, Hui D, Currow DC. Opioids, exertion, and dyspnea: a review of the evidence. *Am J Hosp Palliat Care.* Epub ahead of print: 7 October 2014.

37 Simon ST, Higginson IJ, Booth S *et al.* Benzodiazepines for the relief of breathlessness in advanced malignant and non-malignant diseases in adults. *Cochrane Database Syst Rev.* 2010; (1): CD007354.

38 Repatriation General Hospital. *A Study to Establish whether Further Study of Sertraline in Relieving Severe Breathlessness is Warranted* [clinical trial]. In: Australian New Zealand Clinical Trials Registry (ANZCTR) [website]. ANZCTR identifier: 12608000253303. Camperdown: ANZCTR; 2008. Available at: www.anzctr.org.au/Trial/Registration/TrialReview.aspx?id=82824 (accessed 8 May 2015).

39 Abernethy AP, McDonald CF, Frith PA *et al*. Effect of palliative oxygen versus room air in relief of breathlessness in patients with refractory dyspnoea: a double-blind, randomised controlled trial. *Lancet*. 2010; **376**(9743): 784–93.

40 Currow DC, Agar M, Smith J *et al*. Does palliative home oxygen improve dyspnoea? A consecutive cohort study. *Palliat Med*. 2009; **23**(4): 309–16.

41 Uronis H, McCrory DC, Samsa G *et al*. Symptomatic oxygen for non-hypoxaemic chronic obstructive pulmonary disease. *Cochrane Database Syst Rev*. 2011; (6): CD006429.

42 Uronis HE, Currow DC, McCrory DC *et al*. Oxygen for relief of dyspnoea in mildly- or non-hypoxaemic patients with cancer: a systematic review and meta-analysis. *Br J Cancer*. 2008; **98**(2): 294–9.

43 Johnson MJ, Abernethy AP, Currow DC. The evidence base for oxygen for chronic refractory breathlessness: issues, gaps, and a future work plan. *J Pain Symptom Manage*. 2013; **45**(4): 763–75.

44 McKelvie RS, Moe GW, Cheung A *et al*. The 2011 Canadian Cardiovascular Society heart failure management guidelines update: focus on sleep apnea, renal dysfunction, mechanical circulatory support, and palliative care. *Can J Cardiol*. 2011; **27**(3): 319–38.

45 Bradley TD, Logan AG, Kimoff RJ *et al*. Continuous positive airway pressure for central sleep apnea and heart failure. *N Engl J Med*. 2005; **353**(19): 2025–33.

46 Pozehl B, Duncan K, Hertzog M. The effects of exercise training on fatigue and dyspnea in heart failure. *Eur J Cardiovasc Nurs*. 2008; **7**(2): 127–32.

47 Maddocks M, Gao W, Higginson IJ *et al*. Neuromuscular electrical stimulation for muscle weakness in adults with advanced disease. *Cochrane Database Syst Rev*. 2013; 1: CD009419.

48 Avni T, Leibovici L, Gafter-Gvili A. Iron supplementation for the treatment of chronic heart failure and iron deficiency: systematic review and meta-analysis. *Eur J Heart Fail*. 2012; **14**(4): 423–9.

49 Anker SD, Comin Colet J, Filippatos G *et al*. Ferric carboxymaltose in patients with heart failure and iron deficiency. *N Engl J Med*. 2009; **361**(25): 2436–48.

50 Swedberg K, Young JB, Anand IS *et al*. Treatment of anemia with darbepoetin alfa in systolic heart failure. *N Engl J Med*. 2013; **368**(13): 1210–19.

51 World Health Organization (WHO). *Cancer Pain Relief*. 2nd ed. Geneva: WHO; 1996.

52 Klepstad P, Kaasa S, Jystad A *et al*. Immediate- or sustained-release morphine for dose finding during start of morphine to cancer patients: a randomized, double-blind trial. *Pain*. 2003; **101**(1–2): 193–8.

53 Heerdink ER, Leufkens HG, Herings RM *et al*. NSAIDs associated with increased risk of congestive heart failure in elderly patients taking diuretics. *Arch Intern Med*. 1998; **158**(10): 1108–12.

54 Douglas CA, Moore RK, Leach A *et al*. Modified-release opioids improve pain control

and health-related quality of life in patients with complex cardiac chest pain. *Palliat Med.* 2004; **18**(8): 740–1.

55 Bueno EA, Mamtani R, Frishman WH. Alternative approaches to the medical management of angina pectoris: acupuncture, electrical nerve stimulation, and spinal cord stimulation. *Heart Dis.* 2001; **3**(4): 236–41.

56 Yu W, Maru F, Edner M *et al.* Spinal cord stimulation for refractory angina pectoris: a retrospective analysis of efficacy and cost-benefit. *Coron Artery Dis.* 2004; **15**(1): 31–7.

57 Eldabe S, Raphael J, Thomson S *et al.* The effectiveness and cost-effectiveness of spinal cord stimulation for refractory angina (RASCAL study): study protocol for a pilot randomized controlled trial. *Trials.* 2013; **14**: 57.

58 Tarumi Y, Wilson MP, Szafran O *et al.* Randomized, double-blind, placebo-controlled trial of oral docusate in the management of constipation in hospice patients. *J Pain Symptom Manage.* 2013; **45**(1): 2–13.

59 Nalamachu SR, Pergolizzi J, Taylor R, Jr *et al.* Efficacy and tolerability of subcutaneous methylnaltrexone in patients with advanced illness and opioid-induced constipation: a responder analysis of 2 randomized, placebo-controlled trials. *Pain Pract.* Epub ahead of print: 10 May 2014.

60 Thomas J, Karver S, Cooney GA *et al.* Methylnaltrexone for opioid-induced constipation in advanced illness. *N Engl J Med.* 2008; **358**(22): 2332–43.

61 Clark K, Byfieldt N, Dawe M *et al.* Treating constipation in palliative care: the impact of other factors aside from opioids. *Am J Hosp Palliat Care.* 2012; **29**(2): 122–5.

62 Pasini E, Opasich C, Pastoris O *et al.* Inadequate nutritional intake for daily life activity of clinically stable patients with chronic heart failure. *Am J Cardiol.* 2004; **93**(8 Suppl. 1): 41–3.

63 Aquilani R, Opasich C, Gualco A *et al.* Adequate energy-protein intake is not enough to improve nutritional and metabolic status in muscle-depleted patients with chronic heart failure. *Eur J Heart Fail.* 2008; **10**(11): 1127–35.

64 Anker SD, Steinborn W, Strassburg S. Cardiac cachexia. *Ann Med.* 2004; **36**(7): 518–29.

65 Xander C, Meerpohl JJ, Galandi D *et al.* Pharmacological interventions for pruritus in adult palliative care patients. *Cochrane Database Syst Rev.* 2013; **6**: CD008320.

CHAPTER 6

Supportive care: psychological, social and spiritual aspects

SCOTT MURRAY, MARILYN KENDALL,
MIRIAM JOHNSON AND RICHARD LEHMAN

INTRODUCTION

Patients with heart failure are affected in all aspects of their lives, and patients facing a life-limiting illness should receive attention to their spiritual and psychosocial needs as well as their physical needs.[1] The physical symptoms and disabilities reach out and entangle the way they cope, their emotional buoyancy, their ability to work (and, hence, their finances), and their role in society and within their family. It spreads to their very meaning of life and affects their family and others caring for them. Conversely, social stability and supports, financial security, living accommodation and neighbourhood will affect coping and the ease with which help can be accessed. Supportive care is an essential part of management, but its importance has only recently been emphasised alongside that of medical care. In fact, the perception that the doctor has little or no role in anything other than medication can leave the practitioner feeling helpless and frustrated. A realisation that all healthcare professionals can recognise the multi-domain issues affecting their patients, deal with what they can and refer to appropriate other agencies or professionals as necessary would lead to such supportive care.

Unfortunately, only around 25% of people with non-malignant illnesses are identified for supportive or palliative care before they die.[2] It is important to identify sentinel events, such as emergency admissions, that may indicate that a supportive and palliative care approach is now needed (*see* Figure 6.1). It is equally important to identify the second transition when care for the last days of life (terminal care) is timely.[3] The importance of timely and appropriate access to palliative care and specialist palliative care services is discussed in Chapter 1, 'The need for palliative care in heart failure'. The concepts of 'supportive care' and 'palliative care' are very similar, with the latter being the primary aspect of the former as disease progresses and physical function

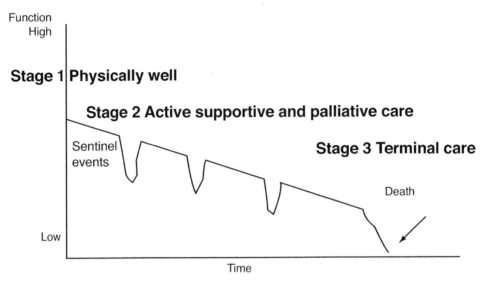

FIGURE 6.1 Caring for people with organ failure: three stages

deteriorates. The term 'supportive care' can be a useful way to introduce the need for a holistic assessment of patient and carer concerns, for patients, carers and clinicians alike, and from which transitions to 'palliative' terminology can be made more easily for those clinicians less used to discussing end-of-life issues.

'Supportive care' is defined by the National Council for Palliative Care as care that

> helps the patient and their family to cope with cancer and treatment of it – from pre-diagnosis, through the process of diagnosis and treatment, to cure, continuing illness or death and bereavement. It helps the patients to maximise the benefits of treatment and to live as well as possible with the effects of the disease. It is given equal priority alongside diagnosis and treatment.[4]

The level and type of support that should be available for adults with cancer is detailed in the National Institute for Clinical Excellence guidelines.[4]

Until the last decade or so, most research studies and health-service developments for people with heart failure focused on medication to reduce mortality and breathlessness, and interventions to prevent hospital readmissions. However, as seen in Chapter 1, a number of studies have sought to gain an understanding of the lived experience of people with heart failure and their informal and professional carers, which can be used to inform the development of a broader range of services that are suitable, accessible and acceptable to patients and carers.[5-12]

In a seminal study in Edinburgh, 20 people with severe heart failure and their carers were interviewed at 3-monthly intervals for up to 1 year.[13] The patients described a pattern of progressive decline, punctuated by episodes of acute deterioration and admission to hospital, growing dependence and an unpredictable terminal phase. Most had been given little information about their illness and prognosis, and gave graphic accounts of uncontrolled symptoms, poor quality of life, and emotional and spiritual distress. Their experience was compared with that of 20 patients dying with lung cancer (summarised in Box 6.1), and it was found they often had very different needs and experiences, a contrast that serves to highlight many of the key issues and debates in the care of heart failure.

BOX 6.1 Summary of the comparative research study[13]

Results

Heart failure patients had a different illness trajectory than the more linear and predictable course of lung cancer patients. In contrast to lung cancer patients, those with cardiac failure had little information about, and a poor understanding of, their condition and prognosis. They were less involved in decision-making. Frustration, progressive losses, social isolation and the stress of balancing and monitoring a complex medication regimen dominated the lives of cardiac failure patients. Heart patients accessed less health-, social and palliative care services, and care was often poorly coordinated.

Conclusions

The experience of dying from these two common conditions was contrasting. Care for people with advanced progressive illnesses is currently prioritised by diagnosis rather than need. Patients, carers and professionals perceive the need to address this inequity. End-of-life care for patients with advanced cardiac failure should be proactive and designed to meet their specific needs.

Although most people talked about the physical aspects of their heart condition, and other illnesses, generally, it was the wider aspects, the ways in which their illnesses had affected their daily and social lives and had compromised their ability to maintain their sense of self, that concerned them most. Many spoke of the 'impossible dream' of living the ordinary life that they used to take for granted, and felt they had been abandoned by the health- and social-care services.

PSYCHOLOGICAL PROBLEMS

Psychological problems are common in chronic illness. Heart failure patients may struggle to cope with increasing debilities and shrinking abilities. Previous ways of coping may be helpful but others less so. Patients may suffer adjustment reactions to progressive losses, which are, in effect, like sequential bereavements. While many patients work through these successfully, just as many people adjust to bereavement or fail to adjust, and anxiety and depression may ensue.

Coping

Such is the resilience of human nature that the majority of patients cope with major health issues without help from healthcare professionals. Of those who do require assistance, probably only a few need the experience and training of clinical psychologists and psychiatrists – the majority managing with the skills of the GP, heart failure nurse, cardiologist or palliative physician. However, it is important to gain an understanding of how the patient usually copes (*see also* Chapter 7, 'Communication in heart failure'). Asking questions such as 'How would you describe yourself before you were ill?', 'What are your strengths?' and 'How have you coped with hard times in the past?' can demonstrate coping strategies learned over many years, and these are likely to be the ones used under stress. This assessment is also useful to remind the patient of the person they are, as this sense can be lost in one who has become overwhelmed by difficulties and ill health. Often during this process, the patient will be able to suggest ways they can help themselves, thus taking back some control over the situation. This is important if there is to be a shared decision-making procedure for treatment. If not done, this may result in a decreasing spiral where the patient feels they are 'lost' in medical management they neither want nor understand in the face of seemingly inevitable deteriorating physical condition. However, it is important to remember that patients do cope differently, and some do not wish for, or are not able to participate in, such joint decision-making. There is no mysterious technique in order to do this – asking the patient usually suffices. 'What is your understanding of your condition?' 'Would you like to know more?' 'What do you think of the treatment plan so far? Would you rather leave that decision to me, or would you like me to discuss it further?'

The way heart failure patients cope with their illness may be mirrored in how they approach understanding their drug treatment. In 2003, 37 patients with heart failure were interviewed and videotaped as part of Health Talk Online.[14] Looking at the heart failure interviews, it became clear that the patients fell into three broad categories.

- The first group seemed to show little understanding of their illness: despite agreeing to a study which mentioned 'heart failure' repeatedly and explicitly, half of them did not realise they had the condition. None of them knew what their drugs were intended to do but did as they were told and left it at that.

- A second group showed greater awareness of their condition and understood part of their drug treatment, and those with access to specialist heart failure nurses found them 'a lifeline'. However, when it came to changes of treatment, they felt that it was best to leave it to their doctors.

- The third (and smallest) group took an active interest in their condition and its treatment and wanted to share in decision-making.

Clearly, some of these differences reflect the educational status of the patients. Some of the differences may also reflect the decision-making style, training and perceived role of the doctors who look after them, or patients' access to specialist nurses. However, this work demonstrates that patients vary widely in their capacity and their desire to be involved in the management of their illness.

A few years earlier, Buetow and colleagues, in Auckland, New Zealand, undertook similar interviews with 62 heart failure patients, specifically examining their coping strategies.[15] They found that the strategies used by patients to cope with their illness as a whole bear a close resemblance to the strategies we have just seen in relation to drug treatment.

- *Avoidance:* Such patients actively avoid information, especially if it is unfavourable. They do not want or accept the need to know.
- *Disavowal:* This appears to be a pre-conscious process. The patients understand the seriousness of the situation, but, to reduce the resultant emotional strain, they dissociate that awareness from its personal reality.
- *Acceptance:* Patients consciously accept the reality of their diagnosis, using understanding and control. Coping is through support from family and friends, drawing on humour and distracting activities.

In this large and representative sample of patients with heart failure, none displayed an outright refusal to acknowledge that anything was the matter with them. However, many patients used some kind of mechanism to downplay the seriousness of their condition, avoid fear and despair, and maintain hope. Therefore, any communication of diagnosis and prognosis has to be done gently, realising that many will find this difficult, as it will not 'fit' with the way they are coping with their illness.

One of the advantages of a coping style that incorporates understanding and control is that it allows practical issues to be addressed with and for the patient. Unless a patient realises what is happening, it is difficult to arrange financial benefits, set up additional care or assess for living aids. Patients are denied the chance for end-of-life planning (legal and financial provision in the settling of affairs, personal choice for place of care) if they do not have a sufficient understanding. Thus, it is imperative that communication is sensitive and skilful, particularly with patients who have less robust coping mechanisms. To do otherwise is to risk pushing a patient who is already struggling to maintain equanimity into depression or anxiety. To avoid the situation by using euphemisms (*see* Chapter 7, 'Communication in heart failure') is to potentially deny a patient their right to know and plan for the future.

Depression

Depression is a common condition in patients with heart failure, with prevalence estimates ranging between 24% and 42%.[16] As with depression in patients with cancer, it often goes undiagnosed and untreated, and the mood disturbance considered to be 'understandable'. Similarly, clinical depression can be difficult to recognise in people with physical illness, as many of the somatic symptoms are present due to the underlying physical illness.

Depression appears to be an important factor in heart failure, as it is independently associated with repeat hospital admissions and a worse prognosis.[17–22]

Heart failure was also noted as a pre-morbid condition in a significant proportion of older patients who committed suicide.[23] Moreover, there is some evidence that depression in the general population is a risk factor for developing heart failure.[18,24] Depression and heart failure share pathophysiological mechanisms and psychosocial issues. It is thought that augmentation of catecholamine release, pro-inflammatory cytokines[24] and platelet activation may be a mechanism whereby depression could make heart failure worse, or even cause it, perhaps by arrhythmias. Depression is also associated with poor social support, which, in turn, is associated with a poorer outcome in heart failure. Depression affects compliance with drug and exercise treatments; thus, it is not surprising to find that one makes the other worse. A prospective study of patients with heart failure showed that patients who lived alone, had a history of alcohol abuse, perceived their medical care to be an economic burden and had poor health status (measured by Kansas City Cardiomyopathy Questionnaire) were more likely to develop depressive symptoms.[25] Each factor was an independent predictor, but if three were present, the incidence of developing depression increased to 69.2%.

Treatment with selective serotonin uptake inhibitors seems to be safe,[26-9] although a Phase III placebo-controlled randomised trial in people with New York Heart Association (NYHA) class II–IV heart failure and major depression failed to show benefit in the primary outcome of the Hamilton Depression Rating Scale or composite cardiovascular status at 12 weeks. A double-blind placebo-controlled pilot study of controlled-release paroxetine on depression and quality of life showed benefit at 12 weeks, but this needs to be confirmed in an adequately powered study.[27] Indeed, there is evidence that their anti-platelet activity has additional effect over and above aspirin.[28] Tricyclic antidepressants are best avoided because of their anticholinergic – hence, pro-arrhythmic – activity.[29] Likewise, venlafaxine has been found to be associated with an increased risk of arrhythmias, although trazadone appears to be safe. Mirtazapine appears to be both safe and effective. Further work should also include longer-term follow-up and investigate the effects of non-pharmacological interventions such as cognitive-behavioural therapy, stress-management techniques,[30] and exercise programmes[31] which seem to be helpful.

It remains to be seen whether treated depression still carries an adverse prognosis in heart failure. Remember that existential distress shares some common symptoms with depression and does not respond to antidepressants.

Anxiety

In the general population, anxiety is often present with depression and may be one of its presenting features. Further, onset of common anxiety constructs has been shown to increase the risk of coronary heart disease, one of the most common causes of heart failure.[32] Anxiety can exacerbate the symptom of breathlessness and superimposed panic attacks can be extremely distressing for patient and carer alike. However, although there is increasing evidence that depression carries a worse prognosis in heart failure, the literature (such as it is) is less clear for anxiety. In a prospective study of 291 patients, Jiang *et al.* found that, although anxiety and depression were both highly correlated in heart failure patients, only depression carried a worse prognosis.[33] Some researchers have concluded that greatly heightened anxiety is not a feature of chronic heart failure,[34] although acknowledge the paucity of the literature – and, indeed, Jiang and colleagues' work was not available at the time of that particular review. It has also been suggested that as natriuretic peptides have shown anxiolytic properties in rodent studies and patients with panic disorder, they may also protect against anxiety in heart failure.[35] Herrmann-Lingen *et al.* showed that the severity of chronic heart failure was significantly related to N-terminal pro-atrial natriuretic peptide levels, poor physical quality of life, vital exhaustion and depression.[35] However, they found no correlation between anxiety and severity of disease. Levels of N-terminal pro-atrial natriuretic peptide were negatively correlated with anxiety and showed an inverse association. They suggested this might be part of a negative feedback loop limiting psychological distress and subsequent adverse autonomic consequences in severe heart failure.

Nevertheless, experience tells us that a level of anxiety – even if it does not often reach anxiety-state severity – is frequently found in patients with chronic disability such as heart failure. Breathlessness, increasing restrictions and worries as to how they will cope concern patients with heart failure. Dysfunctional breathing patterns may be partially alleviated with attention to anxiety management and, occasionally, judicious use of intermediate half-life benzodiazepines, such as lorazepam or lormetazepam, may be helpful. Awareness of unwanted effects is important and is discussed further in Chapter 5, 'Symptom relief for advanced heart failure'. Undisclosed anxieties and concerns may exacerbate the clinical situation, and good communication skills are important (*see* Chapter 7).

Uncertainty and hope

> I don't know how long I've got
>
> Mr K (interviewed by authors)

The course of heart failure, even in its advanced stages, involves a great deal of uncertainty. Uncertainty is generally seen in a negative way: in most life situations, it gives rise to anxiety, and we try to minimise it. However, there is a positive side to uncertainty as well, as Buetow *et al.*[15] point out. They urge GPs to befriend uncertainty in life-threatening illness, because it leaves room for hope. Such hope is not illusory either, because many patients with heart failure do survive for long periods against the odds.

In the Edinburgh study,[13] all the participants spoke of having good days and bad days. However, all found it hard to predict when these would be and, consequently, difficult to know how to plan their lives. Although they wanted to be optimistic about their progress, this was hard to maintain in the face of continual setbacks:

I try to carry on a normal life, but it seems to be one step forward and two back

Mrs KK (interviewed by authors)

I know I won't get better, but I hope it won't get any worse

Mrs BB

People struggled to maintain a normal life while swinging from hope to despair, often in the same day. As such, people often gave parallel accounts of trying to remain positive while also facing the real possibility of dying. An analysis of serial interview studies has revealed that psychological and social distress may be aggravated when there is physical distress such as acute breathlessness in heart failure[36] (*see* Figure 6.2).

SOCIAL PROBLEMS

The practicalities of daily living can become insuperable problems. From the devastation of giving up work, if not already retired, to maintaining the housework, going shopping, doing the gardening and undertaking the more personal issues of bathing and toileting. Financing paid help can be hard if there are insufficient family and friends to help or, indeed, the patient does not wish to put such a burden on those they love. In the UK, there is some non-means-tested state assistance in the form of disability living and attendance allowances. However, these can be daunting to apply for, and, if turned down, the decision can be difficult to appeal against when faced with demoralising bureaucracy, unless there is an advocate for the patient. Due to the difficulties of prognosis and communication, these allowances are often not claimed

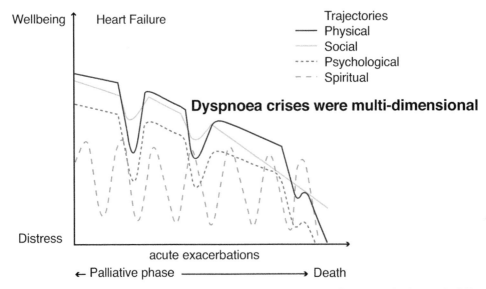

FIGURE 6.2 Patterns of social psychological and spiritual decline towards the end of life in heart failure

under a fast-track system available to patients with cancer, which would mean the money coming through while still timely. Other non-social-security grants are available, but those patients who do not have a well-informed nurse specialist are often disadvantaged in both knowing about them and being able to decipher complicated applications.

The decision to go into nursing-home care can be a deeply distressing one for many, but for those unable to cope, struggling to maintain independence in their own home can also be very frightening. Access to a multi-professional team such as physiotherapy and occupational therapy can be difficult in the community where such resources may be relatively scarce. Funding can also be a problem with regard to what must be paid for by the patient and what will come from the health- or social-services budget. When it is agreed that something – for example, a stairlift – can be provided, it can take time for this provision to be made. In this regard, a hitherto-unmet need is often revealed on referral to the specialist palliative care services.

There does appear to be a relationship between poor social support and hospital admissions and mortality.[37,38] Single marital status correlated with readmission and death in a prospective study of 257 patients.[38] However, marital status on its own does not seem to be the whole story, and the *quality* of a marital relationship has an independent effect on mortality.[39]

Emotional and practical problems were immensely important for the interviewees in the Edinburgh study,[13] but they found it much more difficult to get help in these areas. Things like simply managing the activities of daily living – bathing, dressing, shopping, cooking and cleaning; trying to continue meaningful social interactions by keeping up with holidays, hobbies, and visits to family and friends; dealing with financial matters; and obtaining suitable housing and transport – proved extremely difficult. Most became experts in the logistics of their routine journeys, knowing the barriers, such as hills, they faced and where toilets, and shops they could stop and pretend to look at were. For some, the smallest household job required major planning. Over time, patients lost confidence, making it even less likely that they would go out.

> The tiniest incline is a mountain to me now
>
> Mrs LL (interviewed by authors)

> I'm a home bird now. I like to be near . . . You feel safe when you're at home
>
> Mr T (interviewed by authors)

> I would give the world to be able to go out now
>
> Mr K (interviewed by authors)

Consequently, people's ability to maintain satisfying roles and relationships diminished, and so their self-esteem declined and feelings of dependency grew. Low mood and anxiety were prevalent among both patients and carers as they struggled with the daily grind of living with heart failure:

> I can't do anything else . . . I feel like I'm in prison here with him. I can't go out and each day is just like the last
>
> Carer of Mr Z[40]

A few were able to keep more cheerful, particularly if they had supportive family relationships or were able to hope that things would not get any worse. Humour, a determination not to be beaten, pragmatism and stoicism were all apparent but often-fragile coping strategies, and feelings of uselessness or hopelessness were common. Some patients said their quality of life was so poor that they would welcome death. These feelings were often not admitted to close family for fear of causing distress:

> Frustration – oh yes . . . I see her [his wife] doing things and it makes me feel guilty . . . I just can't do it . . . I find it very, very hard at times.
>
> Mr K (interviewed by authors)

> I think he probably needs a gun . . . if you were a horse, they would shoot you
>
> Carer of Mr N[40]

Perceived ageism emerged, with many patients and carers feeling they had been written off. The frustration felt by GPs that little could be done for these patients, apart from changing the medication, was often conveyed to patients and carers. One patient said:

> I want to be treated like a human being, not a lump of flesh everyone is trying to get rid of
>
> Mr E (interviewed by authors)

There was little evidence of support for informal carers. Partners and children often felt they had no choice about taking on the caring role and extra responsibilities in the changing relationship with their spouse or parent, a role that could continue for many years. Many carers seemed to see the reality of the situation when patients wanted to maintain the pretence of managing well. People without an informal carer faced tremendous difficulties in trying to manage alone in the community. A recent study in primary care identified the reasons why most informal carers for people with long-term conditions are not identified as such and thus fail to be adequately supported.[41]

People with heart failure and their carers described a steadily shrinking social world in which social isolation, co-morbidity and increasing disability were key issues. They spoke with regret of places they could no longer get to, people they could no longer see and hobbies they could no longer pursue. This shrinking world made it difficult for them to maintain any sense of having a meaningful life and worthwhile social interactions.

Clausen *et al.* commented on the Edinburgh study from a social worker's perspective.[42] They highlighted six areas of concern, from the patients' experience, in which social-worker involvement could have made a difference:

(1) loss and dependency, (2) family-centred issues, (3) carer needs, (4) practical tasks, (5) emotional and spiritual struggles and (6) support needs of staff. There is little in the literature regarding the role of the social worker in meeting the needs of patients with anything other than cancer. As a way of addressing some of these issues associated with chronic progressive ill health, Clausen and colleagues called for a return to a holistic 'casework' model of social work rather than 'care management', which only focuses on specific 'identified needs'. They reminded that social workers can provide more than just practical aids and benefits and can also be advocates, counsellors and providers of support.

SPIRITUAL PROBLEMS

Murray *et al.* demonstrated that spiritual issues are important, often the source of unmet need and inextricably linked with all the other problems.[40] These are summarised in Box 6.2.

BOX 6.2 Spiritual needs[40]

- Everyone faced with a serious illness has them.
- An accepted definition used internationally relates to meaning and purpose of life.
- People may or may not use religious vocabulary.
- Such needs may cause distress and increase medical demand.

Patients often looked back at their lives to try to make sense of why this illness had occurred. For some, this involved an element of guilt; one man with heart failure said:

> Maybe this is God turning round and saying 'I'm going to get you back' . . . because I've no' always been a lily-white guy.
>
> Mr HH[40]

Some struggled to find meaning in life, given the restrictions imposed by age, disability and a long-term condition. Often people were admitted to busy hospital wards where spiritual and emotional needs went generally unrecognised:

> The staff are too busy, and you have to learn to look out for yourself. You just have to adapt. I try to hide my grief and be nice to others. That's what they want to see, someone coming in who's cheerful and doesn't complain.
>
> Mr M[40]

Increasing disability altered people's self-image, and proposed solutions, such as using a wheelchair or having help with bathing, could be experienced as depersonalising and degrading, causing spiritual distress:

> She [the occupational therapist] decided I needed boards on the side of my bed, oh aye, that got me. So I said 'Are you going to leave me no dignity at all?' I never saw her again.
>
> Mr E[40]

Topics that are recognised as markers of spiritual distress – such as difficult changes in relationships and social roles, increasing dependence on others for daily needs, feeling isolated and unsupported, lacking self-confidence and feeling frustrated and depressed – formed major themes in the interviews. Some patients, attempting to vocalise feelings of spiritual distress, resisted being labelled 'depressed':

> I'm not depressed . . . not really depressed . . . it's just a low feeling, and it's not a happy feeling, and you just never feel your life's worth anything at times.
>
> Ms J[40]

Hope was difficult to maintain in such circumstances. Many patients spoke of feeling valueless and useless, nothing but a burden to others, and many expressed a wish for death:

> And I said, 'I feel I can't go on. And yet, I don't have the courage, and I never could have the courage, to take my own life. I feel I've reached the end here. But I just wish somebody would come and put me out of my misery.'
>
> Mrs KK[40]

Many people spoke of the strength they drew from being able to maintain their relationships with their families. Opportunities to continue to give and receive love, to feel connected to their social world and to feel useful were highly valued:

> It's not wonderful but I can cope with it, I'm still at home, I'm with my family, I know that they still want me here and I can be of some help to them in looking after the grandchildren. It's a good enough life. It's still worth living, for me.
>
> Mrs A[40]

Those people who were religious found comfort from the support of their church:

> And I get out to the church. My daughter comes every Sunday and takes me, because I can't walk there any more. All my life, even when I was in the army during the war, I would make every effort that I could to get there and that has always given me strength.
>
> Mr K[40]

In the interviews, most GPs said they considered it their role to raise spiritual issues, but felt they lacked the time and training to carry out this role well. They tended to wait for cues from the patients, which were not always forthcoming, especially as patients were not at all sure if dealing with such issues was part of the GP's role.

> But it's not possible with everyone. Some people are very open to it and others are like a brick wall . . . You can't make people talk to you about death and dying.
>
> GP of Mr V[13]

Thus, the spiritual needs of these heart failure patients were characterised throughout by the hopelessness, loss of purpose, isolation and altered self-image associated with chronic illness and disability. These are common to most patients with advanced heart failure, whereas specifically religious issues are probably only significant for a minority.[40] For many people, spiritual needs are not expressed in the language of religion but in terms of the need to maintain a sense of self-worth, to have a useful role in life and retaining an active role with family and friends. The prospect of dying can lead to a deeper level of questioning and searching for meaning and sometimes forgiveness, which can be a lonely struggle going on for months, hidden from health professionals and even from immediate family.

Health professionals may be wary of taking the initiative in exploring these issues, and, indeed, there is some evidence[43] that professionals can sometimes unwittingly contribute to some patients' feelings of worthlessness and loss of dignity. However, adequate time and sensitive use of listening skills, such as empathy and open questioning, can create conditions in which patients and carers feel able to discuss their hopes and fears if they wish. When given the opportunity to discuss spiritual needs with professionals, some patients and carers in the Edinburgh study valued this greatly, both because it validated their concerns and because they felt cherished.[40] Therefore, those most closely involved in looking after patients with advanced heart failure need to be aware of the possibility of spiritual distress, and if they do not feel able to address it themselves, they need to be able to access help from other sources, possibly an experienced chaplain or counsellor.[44,45] There is some evidence to suggest that some unmet existential needs may result in increased needs and service uptake in other dimensions.[46]

Death and dying

Although many had experienced brushes with death during acute episodes, few patients had discussed their preferred place of death or wishes for end-of-life care with professionals.[13,40] Most thought about dying in the context of ageing. Many had made plans with relatives for their funerals and arrangements about money and property. The uncertainty of the prognosis made it difficult for patients and carers to know how imminent death would be, although there was awareness of being 'really ill':

> Sometimes I'm afraid in the morning to go in . . . he's fading away before my eyes . . . It could

be another year or two or it could be another week or two, it could be tomorrow. I don't know.

Carer of Mr N[40]

A final admission to hospital was as likely to be due to a non-cardiac condition as to increasing care needs beyond the capacity of informal carers and community services to cope with. Once admitted, insensitive communication could cause distress:

> They just told us they had a plan . . . they said, we have a plan that if she arrests we will not be resuscitating her. Just as if it was nothing . . . it was terrible

Daughter of Mrs P (interviewed by authors)

Most people reflected on their poor present quality of life:

> I was sitting in a chair all night . . . I would be screaming for air . . . very, very frightening . . . I suppose it's like drowning really.

Mrs A[13]

> It's a life but it's not much of a life. I'm ready for the knacker's yard.

Mrs P[13]

Professionals perceived there was much less support in the community and fewer opportunities for patients to die at home.

A SYSTEM FAILURE

Heart failure patients have huge problems in many areas of their life. At present, many of these appear to be going unheard and being unmet by the current system. Healthcare professionals often do not register these issues, and assistance from the multi-professional team may be lacking. These themes were clearly seen in the Edinburgh study, with heart failure patients often describing negative experiences of hospital admission, with poorly coordinated hospital care, and failure to recognise the involvement and expertise of carers. Seeing different doctors at each hospital appointment caused particular dissatisfaction. Lack of privacy and dignity, with noisy and hectic wards, allowed little time for personalised care.

Primary care contacts were mainly with the GP. There was little planned community support. A few people had developed a long-term relationship with a key professional: a consultant, GP or specialist cardiac nurse. Taking an interest, caring about the person and good communication skills were valued. Specialist palliative care services were not generally involved, and only a minority had access to a specialist cardiac nurse. Social services, financial benefits advice and carer support and respite were largely absent, while information and support from cardiac charities were little used. Care was based on a treatment-focused, medical model. Lack of services, failure to address end-of-life issues and episodes of acute deterioration meant these patients had less opportunity to die at home. One GP stated:

> I'm expecting it [the patient's death] to be something catastrophic, so planning and discussing it isn't really an issue.

> GP of Mrs F[13]

GPs recognised that there were more resources for cancer patients and felt frustrated by their own role, which seemed limited to monitoring and adjusting medication.

SUMMARY

There is an urgent need for the key role of supportive care to be recognised and addressed across the disease trajectory. This should not wait until the situation is so complex that specialist palliative care is involved – rather, cardiology and primary care services should work together to elucidate and tackle the problems. Referral to appropriate agencies and benefits should be routine and done in advance. This could help to prevent emergency hospital admissions due to carer exhaustion and breakdown of the social situation. Clear communication and such advance care planning may also enable the patient to have true choice with regard to preferred place of death, rather than mere rhetoric.

REFERENCES

1 Basta LL. End-of-life medical treatment of older cardiac patients. *Am J Geriatr Cardiol.* 2004; **13**(6): 313–5.
2 Zheng L, Finucane A, Oxenham D *et al.* How good is UK primary care at identifying patients for generalist and specialist palliative care: a mixed methods study. *Eur J Palliat Care,* 2013; **20**(5): 216–22.
3 Boyd K, Worth A, Kendall M *et al.* Making sure services deliver for people with advanced heart failure: a longitudinal qualitative study of patients, family carers, and health professionals. *Palliat Med.* 2009; **23**(8): 767–76.
4 National Institute for Clinical Excellence. *Improving Supportive and Palliative Care for Adults with Cancer: the manual.* London: National Institute for Clinical Excellence; 2004. Available at: www.nice.org.uk/guidance/csgsp/evidence/supportive-and--palliative-care-the-manual-2 (accessed 20 May 2015).
5 Jaarsma T, Beattie JM, Ryder M *et al.* Palliative care in heart failure: a position statement from the palliative care workshop of the Heart Failure Association of the European Society of Cardiology. *Eur J Heart Fail.* 2009; **11**(5): 433–43.
6 Boyd K, Murray SA. Recognising and managing key transitions in end of life care. *BMJ.* 2010; **341**: c4863.
7 Leeming A, Murray SA, Kendall M. The impact of advanced heart failure on social, psychological and existential aspects and personhood. *Eur J Cardiovasc Nurs.* 2014; **13**(2): 162–7.

8   Anderson H, Ward C, Eardley A *et al.* The concerns of patients under palliative care and a heart failure clinic are not being met. *Palliat Med.* 2001; **15**(4): 279–86.

9   Gibbs JS, McCoy AS, Gibbs LM *et al.* Living with and dying from heart failure: the role of palliative care. *Heart.* 2002; 88 (Suppl. 2): ii36–9.

10 Rogers AE, Addington-Hall JM, Abery AJ *et al.* Knowledge and communication difficulties for patients with chronic heart failure: qualitative study. *BMJ.* 2000; **321**(7261): 605–7.

11 Mason B, Epiphaniou E, Nanton V *et al.* Coordination of care for individuals with advanced progressive conditions: a multi-site ethnographic and serial interview study. *Br J Gen Pract.* 2013; **63**(613): e580–8.

12 Hanratty B, Hibbert D, Mair F *et al.* Doctors' perceptions of palliative care for heart failure: focus group study. *BMJ.* 2002; **325**(7364): 581–5.

13 Murray SA, Boyd K, Kendall M *et al.* Dying of lung cancer or cardiac failure: prospective qualitative interview study of patients and their carers in the community. *BMJ.* 2002; **325**(7370): 929–32.

14 http://healthtalkonline.org/

15 Buetow S, Goodyear-Smith F, Coster G. Coping strategies in the self-management of chronic heart failure. *Fam Pract.* 2001; **18**(2): 117–22.

16 Rutledge T, Reis VA, Linke SE *et al.* Depression in heart failure: a meta-analytic review of prevalence, intervention effects, and associations with clinical outcomes. *J Am Coll Cardiol.* 2006; **48**(8): 1527–37.

17 Joynt KE, Whellan DJ, O'Connor CM. Why is depression bad for the failing heart? A review of the mechanistic relationship between depression and heart failure. *J Cardiac Fail.* 2004; **10**(3): 258–71.

18 Pasic J, Levy WC, Sullivan MD. Cytokines in depression and heart failure. *Pychosom Med.* 2003; **65**(2): 181–93.

19 de Denus S, Spinler SA, Jessup M *et al.* History of depression as a predictor of adverse outcomes in patients hospitalized for decompensated heart failure. *Pharmacotherapy.* 2004; **24**(10): 1306–10.

20 Murberg TA, Bru E, Svebak S *et al.* Depressed mood and subjective health symptoms as predictors of mortality in patients with congestive heart failure: a two-years follow-up study. *Int J Psychiat Med.* 1999; **29**(3): 311–26.

21 Jünger J, Schellberg D, Müller-Tasch T *et al.* Depression increasingly predicts mortality in the course of congestive heart failure. *Eur J Heart Fail.* 2005; **7**(2): 261–7.

22 Jiang W, Kuchibhatla M, Clary GL *et al.* Relationship between depressive symptoms and long-term mortality in patients with heart failure. *Am Heart J.* 2007; **154**(1): 102–8.

23 Juurlink DN, Herrmann N, Szalai JP *et al.* Medical illness and the risk of suicide in the elderly. *Arch Intern Med.* 2004; **164**(11): 1179–84.

24 Parissis JT, Adamopoulos S, Rigas A *et al.* Comparison of circulating proinflammatory cytokines and soluble apoptosis mediators in patients with chronic heart failure with versus without symptoms of depression. *Am J Cardiol.* 2004; **94**(10): 1326–8.

25 Havranek EP, Spertus JA, Masoudi FA *et al.* Predictors of the onset of depressive symptoms in patients with heart failure. *J Am Coll Cardiol.* 2004; **44**(12): 2333–8.

26 O'Connor CM, Jiang W, Kuchibhatla M *et al.* Safety and efficacy of sertraline for depression in patients with heart failure: results of the SADHART-CHF (Sertraline

Against Depression and Heart Disease in Chronic Heart Failure) trial. *J Am Coll Cardiol.* 2010; **56**(9): 692–9.

27 Gottlieb SS, Kop WJ, Thomas SA *et al.* A double-blind placebo-controlled pilot study of controlled-release paroxetine on depression and quality of life in chronic heart failure. *Am Heart J.* 2007; **153**(5): 868–73.

28 Serebruany VL, Glassman AH, Malinin AI *et al.* Selective serotonin reuptake inhibitors yield additional antiplatelet protection in patients with congestive heart failure treated with antecedent aspirin. *Eur J Heart Fail.* 2003; **5**(4): 517–21.

29 Alvarez W, Jr, Pickworth KK. Safety of antidepressant drugs in the patient with cardiac disease: a review of the literature. *Pharmacotherapy.* 2003; **23**(6): 754–71.

30 Luskin F, Reitz M, Newll K *et al.* A controlled pilot study of stress management training of elderly patients with congestive heart failure. *Prev Cardiol.* 2002; **5**(4): 168–72.

31 Koukouvou G, Kouidi E, Iacovides A *et al.* Quality of life, psychological and physiological changes following exercise training in patients with chronic heart failure. *J Rehab Med.* 2004; **36**(1): 36–41.

32 Roest AM, Martens EJ, de Jonge P *et al.* Anxiety and risk of incident coronary heart disease: a meta-analysis. *J Am Coll Cardiol.* 2010; **56**(1): 38–46.

33 Jiang W, Kuchibhatila M, Cuffe MS *et al.* Prognostic value of anxiety and depression in patients with chronic heart failure. *Circulation.* 2004; **110**(22): 3452–6.

34 MacMahon KM, Lip GY. Psychological factors in heart failure: a review of the literature. *Arch Intern Med.* 2002; **162**(5): 509–16.

35 Herrmann-Lingen C, Binder L, Klinge M *et al.* High plasma levels of N-terminal pro-atrial natriuretic peptide associated with low anxiety in severe heart failure. *Psychosom Med.* 2003; **65**(4): 517–22.

36 Murray SA, Kendall M, Grant E *et al.* Patterns of social, psychological, and spiritual decline toward the end of life in lung cancer and heart failure. *J Pain Symptom Manage.* 2007; **34**(4): 393–402.

37 Luttik ML, Jaarsma T, Moser D *et al.* The importance and impact of social support on outcomes in patients with heart failure: an overview of the literature. *J Cardiovasc Nurs.* 2005; **20**(3): 162–9.

38 Chin MH, Goldman L. Correlates of early hospital readmission or death in patients with congestive heart failure. *Am J Cardiol.* 1997; **79**(12): 1640–4.

39 Coyne JC, Rohrbaugh MJ, Shoham V *et al.* Prognostic importance of marital quality for survival of congestive heart failure. *Am J Cardiol.* 2001; **88**(5): 526–9.

40 Murray SA, Kendall M, Boyd K *et al.* Exploring the spiritual needs of people dying of lung cancer or heart failure: a prospective qualitative interview study of patients and their carers. *Palliat Med.* 2004; **18**(1): 39–45.

41 Carduff E, Finucane A, Kendall M *et al.* Understanding the barriers to identifying carers of people with advanced illness in primary care: triangulating three data sources. *BMC Fam Pract,* 2014; **15**: 48.

42 Clausen H, Kendall M, Murray S *et al.* Would palliative care patients benefit from social workers' retaining the traditional 'casework' role rather than working as care managers? A prospective serial qualitative interview study. *B J Soc Work.* 2004; **35**(2): 277–85.

43 Fitchett G, Murphy PE, Kim J *et al.* Religious struggle: prevalence, correlates and

mental health risks in diabetic, congestive heart failure, and oncology patients. *Int J Psychiatry Med.* 2004; **34**(2): 179–96.

44 Westlake C, Dracup K. Role of spirituality in adjustment of patients with advanced heart failure. *Prog Cardiovasc Nurs.* 2001; **16**(3): 119–25.

45 Oates L. Providing spiritual care in end-stage heart failure. *Int J Palliat Nurs.* 2004; **10**(10): 485–90.

46 Grant L, Murray SA, Sheikh A. Spiritual dimensions of dying in pluralist societies. *BMJ.* 2010; **341**: c4859.

CHAPTER 7

Communication in heart failure

IAIN LAWRIE AND SUZANNE KITE

Communication is often defined as 'to impart' or 'make known', but its Latin derivation is helpful in emphasizing the 'sharing' of information; *communis* means 'in common'.

Dias *et al.*[1]

INTRODUCTION

Heart failure is affecting more people and affecting them for longer. Medical technology and therapeutics grow apace, and while 'cures' are few and far between, there are an expanding number of treatment options available and long periods with good quality of life are the expectation. While mortality rates from heart failure have fallen,[2,3] morbidity rates may continue to rise due to the growing older population.[2] Thus, there are more and more conversations to be had between doctors and patients discussing the nature and course of heart failure, prognosis, treatment options and patient preferences for end-of-life care. As with other medical developments, the ethical framework and communication skills necessary to permit partnerships with patients have lagged behind the demographics and technology. Very few patients with heart disease have been given the opportunity to discuss end-of-life issues, despite the fact that many have recognised death to be imminent.[4-8] There is also evidence that people with heart failure have less understanding of their illness than do people with in other chronic diseases,[9] perhaps because the term 'heart failure' may not be familiar to patients[5] and consideration of imminent death is largely confined to exacerbations.[10] Many patients with heart failure are ready for, and would welcome, information regarding prognosis, and would like their doctors to start these conversations,[6,11-14] although it should always be recognised that some may not.[8] This would suggest that there is an unmet need in this area of care and also that there is room for improvement in how we communicate with patients with heart failure.

Great strides have been made in communication within oncology through research and dialogue with public, patients and professionals, and there is every reason to hope that the same will become true for heart failure. The need for enhanced communication has been recognised in policy documents,[15] and there is a growing body of work in the healthcare literature.

The term 'communication' encompasses a number of processes and skills. There is a spectrum, from the imparting of information at one end to joint decision-making in complex situations – involving uncertainty and the subtle balancing of benefits, burdens and risks – at the other. Active listening, the ability to elicit patient concerns and to tailor the *sharing* of information and collaborative partnership in decision-making to individual patients are all skills that are necessary and can be learned.[16] *How* we communicate is also as important as what we actually say.

Good communication can lead to identifiable benefits for patients, professionals and healthcare systems. Patients are given the opportunity to take a more active role in the management of their illness through being better informed and being included in decision-making. This can have a positive effect on patients[17,18] and can lead to enhanced patient and carer satisfaction with care. Healthcare staff also benefit, as improved communication with patients contributes to a more open relationship in which responsibilities and decisions are shared. This can lead to improved clinical care and professional well-being.[19] Better-informed patients, who are more involved in their own care, have also been shown to have improved compliance with treatment regimens, which, in turn, results in decreased rates of readmission to hospital.[18,20,21] Such effects have positive ramifications for both health professionals and the healthcare system. Conversely, lack of open communication can lead to a substandard level of care.[22]

In this chapter, we present an overview of communication in heart failure. We examine what patients need and wish to know, and explore some of the potential barriers to effective communication for this patient group. We then review various strategies that have been tried to improve communication with heart failure patients and reflect on their effectiveness. Learning points that may be transferred from experience in oncology and palliative care are considered, along with suggestions for how effective communication skills can be learned. Advance care planning (ACP) in heart failure is also examined. Finally, ways forward for communication in specific situations common in heart failure care are explored.

WHAT MIGHT NEED TO BE COMMUNICATED?

Heart failure is a complex diagnosis with an uncertain and non-uniform pathway of illness.[23] Many aspects require patient involvement and further discussion. Explanation about the nature of the condition, what may have caused it, the physical changes that have occurred and the symptoms such changes might bring about forms part of the communication process. Patients often lack clear understanding of these aspects of their illness.[24-7] Discussion of symptoms leads to exploration of the effects and limitations such symptoms may have on their lives. Patients may want to know what management strategies are available, including both pharmacological and non-pharmacological therapies, and about the potential burdens or side effects of treatment. This is especially true for cardiac transplantation. Discussion of prognosis is important so that patients and their families can make plans, but in a way that preserves hope, when possible. However, patients may not ask about prognosis unprompted and may not be aware of the management options available to them.[28] End-of-life care planning also involves discussion of more difficult topics, such as changing the emphasis of treatment; starting or stopping treatment, including implantable cardiovertor defibrillators (ICDs); future care planning; resuscitation status; and 'do not attempt cardiopulmonary resuscitation' (DNACPR) orders and advance decisions to refuse treatment. All these topics are difficult for both patient and professional to discuss and require sensitivity in communication.

WHAT DO WE KNOW ABOUT WHAT PATIENTS WANT?

I think the best physician is the one who has the providence to tell to the patients according to his knowledge the present situation, what has happened before, and what is going to happen in the future.

Hippocrates (470–410 BC) (Beng[29])

Often, there can be a chasm between what professionals *think* their patients want to know and what patients and their carers *actually* want to know, or not know. However, it is clear that many patients and their carers wish for more information than professionals estimate.[30] In a study by Formiga *et al.*,[31] 64% of patients were aware of the chronic and progressive nature of their condition, but McCarthy and colleagues[32] reported that nearly half of patients in their study had been unable to get all the information they wanted.

Nurses involved in the care of patients with heart failure have reported that professionals tend to focus the care they provide for this group of patients on symptom control and drug management.[33] However, patients and carers want a more holistic approach to their care, addressing information needs and psychosocial concerns,[34] as well as the physical aspects of their illness.

Much of the literature suggests that patients want open and honest discussions, often repeated,[13] with the professionals involved in their care,[13,14,35,36] and covering all aspects of their illness, both positive and negative. They want information on and support with how to achieve a good quality of life during their illness[37] and education regarding their medication and treatment.

Cardiopulmonary resuscitation (CPR) is an issue that patients may have considered and wish to talk about. However, it may not be discussed, even in conversations around future care planning.[38] Professionals should approach discussion of resuscitation to determine to what extent the patient wishes to be involved in making such decisions.[39]

Communication regarding prognosis can be difficult, and many patients with advanced disease can be overly optimistic about their prognosis.[40,41] In one study, many more professionals than patients or carers believed that discussions regarding prognosis had already taken place,[7,42] suggesting that communication had not been effective. Such discussions are important to patients, particularly as their illness progresses and they have a limited time left to live.[42]

Nevertheless, not all patients want frank and open discussion, and this wish should be respected. Some are not open to receiving specific prognostic information, preferring to avoid receiving bad news.[6,43,44] This was demonstrated by a study that found that 100% of patients wanted the professionals caring for them to be honest but, at the same time, 91% also wanted them to maintain hope or be optimistic.[43]

> Patients with disabling, progressive illnesses expect active care, but they also seek comfort, control and dignity.
>
> Murray *et al.*[45]

POTENTIAL BARRIERS TO COMMUNICATION

> [C]ommunication is only effective when the patient understands what the clinician has said.
>
> Fried *et al.*[42]

Effective communication goes beyond *what* is said and what is done during an encounter with a patient. A great many factors can have a detrimental effect on the quality of the experience and its effectiveness. Such factors are often referred to as 'barriers' to communication and can be described across a number of domains: patient, disease, professional and system.

Patient-related factors

There are a number of potential barriers to communication in patients with heart failure. Limited exercise tolerance, fatigue, breathlessness and medical co-morbidities are all prevalent in this patient group and can seriously restrict the patient's ability to both attend and actively participate in outpatient appointments.[11] Breathlessness and fatigue limit the patient's ability to tell their story, express their concerns and ask questions. Patients with heart failure tend to be older, and co-morbid conditions, such as dementia, poor eyesight and hearing difficulties, are all more common in this group.[46]

Psychosocial functioning is often impaired in patients with heart failure[47,48] and is described more fully in Chapter 6, 'Supportive care: psychological, social and spiritual aspects'. Depression can impair decision-making for a number of reasons, from the forming of negative inferences to the reduced ability to think clearly, logically and constructively in complex situations. A high incidence of major depression (17%–26%) has been reported among people with chronic heart failure.[49,50] Minor depression is also common, being present in almost a third of patients.[50] Increased mortality among patients with heart failure who are depressed has been documented.[49-52] Patients with heart failure with significantly altered mood also tend to display reduced compliance with disease management,[53-5] consult their doctor more often and have more frequent readmissions to hospital.[50] Depression can persist or worsen following hospital discharge.[49,56,57] Several characteristics of depressed mood (e.g. fatigue, inability to concentrate, hopelessness, lack of social interaction, paucity of speech) serve to confound the communication process and decrease the involvement of the patient in their care. Such symptoms, common in heart failure, may mask depression, and good communication skills are required both to diagnose and to manage depression.

The lack of a common language used by patients, carers and professionals is in itself a barrier to effective communication. All must be able to understand not only what is said but also the associated meanings. As mentioned, the term 'heart failure' is often not used by patients.[5] This may be because it conjures up images of a part of their body that is gradually weakening, which they find difficult to cope with. The term itself can be very emotive; one 'fails' an exam or is in a marriage that fails, for example. In addition, the term 'heart' is central to our sense of self, our seat of emotion, our being and life itself. Therefore, it is understandable that patients can avoid using the label 'heart failure', and professionals need to be aware of this when discussing diagnosis. Alternatively, avoidance of the term may reflect the fact that they have not received sufficient information or explanation to be able to understand their illness properly.

Patients may also attribute a lack of information and discussion to reluctance by the professional to give them too much or inappropriate information.[11] Cues from the patient may also be subtle or missing. For example, patients attending outpatient clinics may prioritise the information they pass on to the professional, as they realise that such visits are often limited by time and, indeed, the professional agenda is one of 'balancing and monitoring' medication and physical symptoms.[58,59] Patients may not volunteer information or opinion, feeling that to express their own views or wishes may seem ungracious in some way. They may feel that the cardiologist has put so much effort into caring for them and they do not know how to say that they do not want a particular treatment. However, patients do often offer verbal and non-verbal cues during a consultation that may indicate a desire to discuss sensitive issues.[23] Unfortunately, even if the patient explicitly requests information or tries to initiate such discussions, some doctors still find difficulty in engaging.[23] This unconscious negotiation, whereby the patient tacitly accepts the professional agenda, can lead to a less-than-ideal exchange of information.[60]

Disease-related factors

Other symptoms associated with cardiac insufficiency also affect communication. Confusion and poor short-term memory can have a significant impact on the ability to communicate effectively with friends, carers and professionals.[11] Patients with heart failure may have difficulty in retaining information,[61] which inhibits the process of building on previous encounters, developing discussions and assimilating information into a coherent overview of their disease, treatment and prognosis. In turn, this makes discussion about patients' wishes regarding future care more difficult and can be a barrier to informed decision-making.

The very variable and unpredictable course of the disease also poses significant challenges.[34,62] The relapsing–remitting nature of heart failure means that professionals often find it difficult to identify appropriate stages at which to discuss certain management options or approach changes to the direction of care or prognosis.[23] The possibility of death, especially sudden death, is often not discussed openly. In New York Heart Association (NYHA) class II heart failure, annual mortality is estimated at 5%–15%, but 50%–80% of these patients can die suddenly.[63-5] At later stages of the disease (NYHA class IV), the annual mortality is 30%–70%, yet only 5%–30% die suddenly.[66] Although these data may help to focus information more accurately in this difficult patient group, individuals often do not relate their situation to statistics and can interpret statistics in a number of ways.

Professional-related factors

Professionals cannot agree on a single definition of heart failure and, as a result, can be reluctant to use the term[5] or find it very difficult to explain the diagnosis to the patient.[27] It can be particularly difficult to translate extensive knowledge about such a complex pathophysiological process into language appropriate for individual patients, and doctors may feel that the term 'heart failure' may reflect a higher degree of risk than they wish to convey.[67] Further, doctors can believe that patients expect too much certainty, particularly with prognosis[68,69] and, being unable to provide this, can avoid communicating key information entirely. The disease is progressive and the course unpredictable, and professionals, through the inevitable inability to foresee deteriorations in their patients' illness trajectories, can feel impotent.

The professional may also see their role as one solely of monitoring medical treatment and may feel uncomfortable about extending the relationship into a more equal one of the sharing of information and decision-making. This may be a result of the traditional model of undergraduate training in history taking and examination, in which the focus has been on making a diagnosis and formulating a treatment plan. Recently, this approach has been questioned, and this has resulted in the development of the extended Calgary–Cambridge model,[70,71] which outlines and structures the skills that have been shown by research and theory to aid doctor–patient communication. In this model, history taking and examination are wholly integrated with forming a relationship with the patient, so that joint decision-making can occur. Although relatively well developed in primary care, it is now beginning to form the basis of consultation-skills training in some medical schools.[72] It is encouraging that future professionals may not only consider communication to be their job but also that *how* they discuss the problem with the patient is of equal importance to the medical or surgical management of that problem. The past few decades have seen a marked change in the doctor–patient relationship, with paternalism largely having been replaced with a number of models in which respect for patient autonomy is central.[73] Two of the main models are the client-provider and the partnership. The former is more appropriate for well patients seeking specific procedures; the role of the doctor is technician and the patient is the decision-making client. The partnership model recognises the unique skills and perspectives of both patient and physician working together towards optimal care for the individual, and does require significant investment by the patient in time and understanding. Not all frail palliative care patients can meet the demands of the partnership model at all times and, in these situations, best-interest considerations will help the doctor make decisions for the patient based on their known preferences and goals.[74] The range of coexisting models of the doctor–patient relationship raises the possibility of misunderstanding between any particular patient and their doctor regarding which model is desired and which is in operation. Establishing mutual expectations is an important element of good communication.

Health professionals have their own attitudes and emotions to contend with. Peter Kaye's work[75] in the field of breaking bad news can be generalised more widely in clinical practice. He describes how doctors can experience feelings of incompetence, embarrassment, and of being 'powerless' and 'failing' the patient, as well as being reminded of their human vulnerability. They may feel ill-prepared for such discussions[76] or that discussing issues around the end-of-life is an admission of failure;[77] they may feel awkward about showing emotion or sympathy, seen by some as anathema to their 'clinical' role; they may fear being blamed by patients or carers for the progression of the patient's illness and feel powerless at not being able to offer readycures. Some may fear unleashing an emotional reaction from the patient or their carers, which they will find hard to manage, or fear that distress itself may further harm the patient. Professionals can prefer to shield the patient from bad news, perhaps in an attempt to prevent causing distress or damaging hope.[27,45,67] If an earlier patient consultation has not occurred as the professional would have liked or has been awkward, subsequent interactions with other patients may be negatively affected.[78] All these emotions and thoughts, engendered in the professional in what can be stressful situations,[79,80] can inhibit open communication between patient and professional.

The reality is that heart failure is associated with very debilitating symptoms, social problems and suffering. Professionals try to balance providing patients with information with a desire to maintain their hope[81-3] in a condition in which the limitations and burdens of disease are high and the prognosis far from certain.

System-related factors

The 'mechanics' of the healthcare system also influence quality of communication for patients and carers. Care of patients with heart failure has been described as uncoordinated,[77,84] with lack of continuity of care and community support contributing to repeated admissions and discharges between hospital and community sectors. When patients are admitted to hospital, they are not necessarily looked after by the same team of professionals as before, and medical records can be missing or their receipt delayed. A bias towards cancer within palliative care also remains, and provision for patients with non-malignant diseases can be variable.[77]

An absence of coherent, planned patient care in the community, especially for those in the terminal stages of their disease, coupled with a lack of specialist support for general practitioners, represents a barrier to communication on a wider scale:

> [B]ecause the consultants are managing patients when they're on the wards and the general practitioners are trying to manage them at home, they're falling between two stools, and that seems to me to be a real problem.
>
> Cardiologist (Hanratty *et al.*[84])

Both patients and professionals have identified that time constraints limit communication opportunities.[58,59,75] If time is too limited, patients' ideas, concerns and expectations cannot be fully explored, and patients may be reluctant to 'bother the busy doctor'. Busy cardiology clinics, at which 10-minute appointments are allocated, are not appropriate for the cardiologist to deal with the complexities of heart failure. Attention to the set-up and running of clinics, with increasing use of heart failure nurse specialists and facilities where discussions may be held in private, are helpful strategies. Table 7.1 summarises the potential barriers to communication.

LESSONS LEARNED IN COMMUNICATION FROM OTHER AREAS OF MEDICINE

Much of the work in communication in hospital medicine and healthcare over the past half-century has been in the field of oncology. Until the 1970s, cancer patients in the UK were rarely informed of their prognosis and had little opportunity to be involved in decision-making regarding their management.[85] On the grounds that treatment options were limited and the prognosis, even with such treatment, was poor, it was considered cruel to burden patients with this information. However, pioneering oncologists and palliative care physicians realised that, far from reducing suffering, this approach added to patient and carer distress and isolation, and, increasingly, doctors not only gave patients more information[86–8] but also involved them more as partners in decision-making.

Early work in communication looked at how best to break bad news. Simple, step-by-step approaches were developed, and communication skills teaching is now a core component of most undergraduate medical curricula and many training programmes for other health professionals. Indeed, the central role of good communication in the provision of effective healthcare has been

TABLE 7.1 Barriers to communication

Type of barrier	Barriers
Patient and disease related	• Difficulty in attending and participating in clinic appointments due to symptoms
	• Co-morbidities such as dementia, poor eyesight and hearing
	• Depression
	• Lack of 'common language'
	• Tacit acceptance of professional agenda
	• Cognitive impairment
	• Relapsing–remitting nature of disease
	• Difficulty with prognosis
Professional related	• No agreed single definition of the disease
	• Perception that patients want prognostic certainty
	• See role solely as monitoring medical treatment
	• Do not want to upset patients
	• Feeling of powerlessness
System related	• Poorly coordinated care, especially between primary and secondary care
	• Lack of planning and continuity of care
	• Time constraints

recognised at a national level, with such skills training being recognised in policy documents.[89]

Breaking bad news is just one aspect of communication in cancer care; skills are also required in communicating prognosis, giving complex information, obtaining informed consent, discussions with relatives, eliciting and managing psychosocial concerns, and coping with the emotions of both patients and carers.

More recently, the communication literature has addressed the area of communication and management of risk and uncertainty, not just in oncology but also in many other areas of medicine. A growing body of work exists regarding how patients make health decisions and what they need, want and expect from health professionals. There is a move away from patients being seen as passive recipients of information towards a new role as informed and involved partners in shared decision-making.

The key messages arising from the work in oncology can be generalised to other fields. The importance of telling patients the truth at a pace, and to a level, tailored to their individual need is well established. Such information is necessary for patients to make informed choices about treatment, their personal lives and how and where they spend their time. Informing patients sensitively, empathetically and honestly respects their autonomy and helps to build the trusting professional relationships necessary at a time of crisis. Conversely, withholding information tends to compound fear and anxiety, while removing the basis of trust, leaving patients scared and isolated. The vast majority of patients want to be well informed but not all do. A significant minority would prefer to leave 'bad news' for now and face the consequences later, and it usually transpires that this is an enduring, lifelong coping strategy that may have served them well. Such situations require even greater sensitivity in negotiating the pace and timing at which information is shared. It should not be assumed that professionals 'instinctively' know how much information and how great a role in decision-making individual patients want at any particular time. Preferences can and do fluctuate over time. It is important for professionals to question their assumptions, particularly if they are making generalisations based on gender, age, culture or educational background, as these are unreliable predictors. On the whole, younger patients want more information and to be more involved in decision-making[90] but so may certain older individuals. An individual approach is needed, and the best approach is to talk with the patient.

However, such skills in sensitive and empathic communication and negotiation require training and support. The day-to-day barriers of time pressures and lack of privacy, combined with the emotionally demanding nature of the work, can erode good practice in even the most skilled. End-of-life discussions challenge us all, exposing our own beliefs and fears about death and dying. Addressing end-of-life concerns in others may be very discomforting. Communication skills training offers the opportunity to step back and confront one's own professional and personal insecurities, while learning a structured approach to communication, and it has been shown to lead to improved attitudes, confidence and skills in participants.[90-3]

Oncologists and palliative care specialists have learned to reflect on the language they use to avoid ambiguity. For instance, terms such as 'bladder warts', 'growths', 'tumours', 'cure of local disease', 'progressing' and even 'mischief' have all been found to be misleading (deliberately or otherwise) and are best avoided.

Step-by-step models of sharing bad news have been developed.[75,94] Such models emphasise the need to pace discussions, so that difficult information can be conveyed with the patient feeling that they have some control over the direction of the conversation and are not overwhelmed. Preparatory steps include finding a suitable location that affords some privacy and freedom from interruptions; ensuring that the appropriate people are present, especially a friend or family member if the patient wishes; having the necessary notes and investigation results available; and clarifying the purpose of the discussion and the patient's understanding of what has led up to this point. Such preparation often affords the patient a 'warning shot' of what is to come and, as the doctor starts to deliver the news, more signals may be given to enable the patient to centre themselves. An example might be:

Doctor: Your GP asked you to come to clinic because your symptoms were

causing concern. Your recent tests have shown why you have been feeling so tired. Would you like me to explain the results?
Patient nods.
Doctor: I'm afraid to say that it is serious . . .
Patient looks away . . . doctor pauses . . .
Doctor: Would you like me to go on?
Patient: I've got cancer haven't I?
Doctor: I'm sorry to say that, yes, the results did show cancer.

This brief excerpt illustrates the use of a number of warning shots – using words and phrases such as 'of concern' and 'serious' – and also how the doctor uses cues from the patient to pace the giving of information. Subsequently, the doctor allows the patient time to start absorbing the information and encourages them to express their feelings and concerns. When the patient is ready, the discussion moves on to addressing these concerns and discussing the next step, the management plan. Again, the patient is encouraged to ask questions, their understanding of the situation is checked and the outcome of the consultation summarised. An offer would then be made for a further opportunity to continue the discussion and a point of contact established for concerns arising in the meantime. Some services offer an audiotape or written summary of the conversation. A summary of the discussion must be recorded in the patient notes and communicated to the other key healthcare professionals involved in immediate patient care, such as the general practitioner. This approach highlights how communication is a *process* rather than a one-off event.

The importance of communication with family members or close friends of the patient is fundamental to palliative care. Such discussions must be with the permission of competent patients. Sometimes, family members insist on information being withheld from the patient for various reasons but usually in an attempt to protect the patient from distress. Experience has shown that this is nearly always the 'wrong' thing to do. While acknowledging the insights of family members, healthcare professionals can tactfully help family to see that such collusion can add to the patient's distress. Patients usually pick up on non-verbal cues and can lose trust in their carers, are prevented from making informed choices, will often be aware of the progress of their physical condition and will expect answers sooner or later.

HOW TO LEARN COMMUNICATION SKILLS

Communication skills are not an optional add-on extra; without appropriate communication skills, our knowledge and intellectual efforts are easily wasted.

Silverman *et al.*[71]

The 'innate' skills of healthcare professionals do not seem to be sufficient to identify patient concerns, picking up on only about 40% of the issues of importance to patients,[95,96] largely physical symptoms. Communication skills training can help professionals to identify concerns and help patients and carers to find strategies to resolve problems or to adapt to them, with the aim of reducing emotional and physical distress.

Different approaches to teaching communication skills in cancer care have evolved. The format of a 2- to 3-day small-group, workshop-based course, sometimes residential and often multi-professional, is common. Such courses, which use interaction and reflection as well as practise and refining of skills with immediate feedback in a supportive environment, became a popular option for those specialising in cancer and palliative care in the 1990s. The Maguire approach to acquiring communication skills[81] encourages participants to recognise barriers to disclosure of concerns and to overcome them. Participants are shown how to pick up and respond to cues, and to encourage patients to talk about their perceptions and emotional responses to events. The use of tentative, educated guesses to uncover undisclosed concerns and the use of summarising and checking patient understanding are also taught. Skills learned are applied to differing scenarios such as anger, denial, collusion and patients who are withdrawn.

Some evaluations of the efficacy of such courses have produced inconclusive results,[97] partly as a result of the difficulty in identifying suitable outcome measures in such a complex field with many interacting variables. However, some are more encouraging regarding the benefits of such training,[98,99] reporting an increase in patient disclosures following training and maintenance of this improvement at six months.[99] Practically, the main drawback to such courses is they are both time and labour intensive, with too few qualified trainers to meet current demand for training. Other methods of teaching communication skills, such as shorter interactive courses with larger groups, supervision in clinical practice, informal apprenticeship and shadowing, and lecture-based formats, are widespread. However, formal evaluation of efficacy is often lacking for the reasons already stated. It is also thought that training that does not include some form of 'safe skills practice' – that is, role play, observation or feedback – merely raises awareness rather than brings about a change in practice. It is hoped that changes to medical undergraduate curricula with regard to communication skills training will make a positive difference to clinicians' practice in the future.

WHAT STRATEGIES HAVE BEEN TRIED REGARDING COMMUNICATION IN HEART FAILURE?

Good communication encompasses the availability of clear, 'readable' information at the right time and in the right place; the application of such information through education; and the knowledge, skills and attitudes to facilitate decision-making for the individual patient. Information and education are largely beyond the scope of this chapter. However, it should be noted that formal education and support interventions extending beyond the hospital setting can reduce adverse clinical outcomes and costs for patients with heart failure.[100] A comprehensive review of education and heart failure is available.[101]

The emerging literature in communication and heart failure is based largely on research of patient perceptions and concerns and is more suggestive of strategies to be tried rather than descriptive or evaluative of current practice. It is a dynamic field of enquiry, and some of the themes relating to language, supporting structures, coping strategies and communication of risk will be explored here.

Language

Language is fundamental to good communication, which is about finding out which words help and which ones hinder. Some professionals seem to have an 'innate' ability to do this well, while most learn from experience and feedback. Although colleagues may be able to help with feedback, asking patients which words they use and find helpful or otherwise is essential to hear themes that relate to conceptions of disease, interpretation of symptoms and effect on everyday life.

We have already mentioned that patients may not recognise the term 'heart failure' or use it in relation to themselves, that some doctors may also avoid the term because of its negative connotations,[5,102] as well as that 'heart' is an emotive word for people and that the use of the word 'failure' usually connotes negative experiences within our culture. Patients do use very negative terms in explaining their conceptions of their illness, 'such as "dead", "rubbish", "diseased", "gone completely", or "scarred tissue" to describe the condition of their heart'.[103] Whether such terms have originated from doctors or have been thought of by patients is unclear. Patients can also pick up terms from other patients while waiting to see the professional or after a consultation. Such 'second-hand' knowledge may not relate to their disease state and could be misleading to them.

Choice of language can create a dilemma for professionals. The use of medical terms may ensure openness within the consultation but can result in negative emotions when used.[67,102,104] To avoid such reactions, Tayler and Ogden go on to explain that professionals may resort to the use of euphemisms, which they may feel to be 'more neutral and less emotive'.[67] Their research, carried out among patients with heart failure in primary care, found that this appeared to be borne out in clinical practice. Use of the term 'heart failure' resulted in increased levels of anxiety and depression among patients, and they viewed their illness as being more serious. It may be that the professional tailors the language they use to specific situations; but the use of euphemisms carries its own difficulties, and it may be one of the reasons why patients with heart failure have less opportunity for end-of-life planning and less understanding of their condition compared with those dying of lung cancer, for example. Indeed, the use of euphemisms has been discouraged in the field of oncology because of this problem.

Heart failure is a devastating experience, and the realities of patients need to be respected. Yet, at times, a lack of professional sensitivity can also hinder communication, as this quotation from a general practitioner to a patient illustrates: 'You're paddling downstream to Niagara'.[45] This comment is telling, because patients may themselves use metaphors, often relating to wind and water, in describing their experience of heart failure.[105] In her qualitative study, Zambroski outlined how patients described different phases of their illness in terms of 'experiencing turbulence, navigating, and finding safe harbour' and symptoms related to 'too much water' and 'not enough wind'.[105] The understanding of heart failure in terms of impact on everyday life is evident in many qualitative studies, for example:

> [I]t's hard to put into words in't, but what I understand about it is it puts me out of breath and I can't walk and can't do owt.
>
> Male, age 70 years (Horne[103])

Another group examined patient descriptors of breathlessness in heart failure, finding three dominant experiences of breathlessness – 'every day', 'worsening' and 'uncontrollable' – descriptions quite distinct from medical terminology.[106] Research with patients to identify a common language with their professional carers is at an early stage, but it promises to offer a constructive basis for dialogue.

A coordinated service framework

A coordinated service framework is necessary to facilitate good communication.[84] Such a service framework needs to describe how different professionals communicate with patients and each other and also who will take responsibility for the communication of specific aspects of care, including an assessment of psychosocial concerns. This is likely to differ from place to place, depending on local resources and personnel. In most localities, though, it should be possible to identify a 'key worker' to take the lead in coordinating care across care settings (especially hospital to home). Increasingly, this coordinating role is being taken by heart failure clinical nurse specialists. However, general practitioners, district nurses, cardiologists, medicine-for-older-people physicians and specialist palliative care team members may be appropriate practitioners for certain individuals in certain places. As many patients experience difficulty in getting to hospital appointments, mechanisms for home assessments or telephone consultations (if appropriate) should be in place. A key aspect of this collaborative approach to communication with and about patients with heart failure is ensuring that consistent information is discussed and shared.[107]

Coping mechanisms in the self-management of heart failure

Coping mechanisms in the self-management of heart failure are discussed in Chapter 6. An understanding of different models of coping is particularly important to communication in the field of chronic illnesses such as heart failure that are associated with progressive symptoms that seriously limit everyday life and patient choices. When giving patients news that will negatively affect their hopes and quality of life, it is vital to be able to understand and to convey some means by which patients and their carers may be able to absorb this information and 're-centre' themselves in the light of the new information.

Everyday clinical conversations

Everyday clinical conversations happening in the routine process of care can be a vehicle for complex discussions, including foregoing life support.[35] Such conversations, progressing through patient perception of the situation to thoughts about diagnosis, prognosis and possible treatments, may be demanding and difficult for sick patients but appear to be well tolerated, even valued, particularly by most (but not all) patients if a family member is present.[35]

> Within 10–20 minutes of conversation most patients seemed to be ready to talk about fundamental questions of life and death. It was also quite easy to get an idea of both the patient's values and his or her understanding of medical issues. For example, their knowledge about CPR was often very poor . . . no one said that they had been troubled by the conversation itself. Many patients approved. They also emphasised that it is the doctors' duty to give such information to their patients.
>
> Löfmark and Nilstun[35]

Such conversations also help to clarify personal treatment goals for individual patients and wishes for the future direction of care and involvement of those close to the patient in decision-making.[38] Others advocate the taking of an ethics history as part of a routine clerking, including attitudes towards, and preferences for, end-of-life care, preferred model for participation in decision-making, the existence of advance directives and preferences for relatives to receive information.[108]

More information and discourses from the everyday practice of clinical nurse specialists working with patients with heart failure would be informative. Each will be learning and adapting strategies from which other professionals could learn. Mike Connolly, nurse consultant in palliative care and national clinical lead of The Heart Improvement Programme, provides some of this richness in a personal account of his own practice. He highlights the fundamental principles of 'patient-centred care', not least that the patient is 'an untapped source of solutions and ways forward' and that patients can be greatly empowered by approaches that place them firmly in control of their care. He works by negotiation when, first, a patient agrees to explore their situation and second, when both patient and nurse work together to find solutions. This is illustrated in the following dialogue:

> Of course I can't fix all your problems. I may actually not be able to help at all but I'd like to try if you want me to. It may be that if we put our two heads together we can make some sense of your situation and get you back to coping and feeling something like yourself again.
>
> Connolly (personal account to editors, 2005)

Such an approach requires time (40 minutes plus). Connolly advocates starting with an exploration of what the patient perceives their strengths to be and how they have coped with previous difficulties, before progressing to current problems and any thoughts the patient might have about addressing these problems. He advises against starting with a formal medical history, as this might set a medical agenda and be a less effective use of time if the aim of the session is to explore psychosocial concerns and coping mechanisms. Connolly describes the single most useful question he has learned as 'Who were you before you were ill?', admitting that it takes many patients by surprise but can be a valuable tool for uncovering hopes, strengths, coping styles and self-esteem. Subsequent listing of current problems often helps patients to recognise why they can feel so overwhelmed and can be a springboard for moving forward to identify realistic goals and actions.

Communication of risk and uncertainty

Communication of risk and uncertainty is a current focus of communication research. Getting communication of risk and uncertainty right is crucial to partnership models of healthcare. Currently, it is beset with difficulties. Patients need to be as informed as possible for partnerships to be real. However, little is known about how to present risk and to communicate and live with uncertainty as positively as possible. Risk information can be presented in many ways, including absolute risk, relative risk, percentages, odds and fractions, often all in the same consultation.[46] This is confounded by the fact that the data are usually derived from clinical trials with strict inclusion criteria, often excluding the very group of patients to which the individual patient belongs. Different mathematical representations may be understood to a lesser or greater extent than others, and with wide variance between individuals. There is also the question of 'Risk of what?'. Doctors are likely to be focusing on risk of mortality and morbidity, whereas the patient's focus may be on the likelihood of treatment restoring quality of life.[109] This very much represents work in progress, but research in this area may yield practically useful results.

Some patients welcome the opportunity to discuss and plan for their future care in advance. This may be the case at any stage of illness; however, there is an added urgency when the patient's underlying disease is progressing through the disease-modifying medical treatments that are available. The importance of ACP for patients with heart failure has been emphasised through the publication of guidelines.[110-13] However, ACP discussions, which aim to agree goals, preferences and priorities of care, can be difficult for both patients and professionals and are often avoided by doctors, perhaps due to the uncertain disease trajectory,[114] but, when they happen, often take place far too late to be of any meaningful or practical benefit for the patient or those who care for them.[23]

Early preparation and planning for the future is an important element of care.[23] However, discussing the wide range of issues related to ACP can be time-consuming,[115] which may be a reason why such areas are often avoided during outpatient consultations. It may be appropriate, though, to address individual concerns adequately over a number of appointments to build up a comprehensive advance care plan for each patient. Discussions, and the decisions made as a result, should be clearly documented, regularly reviewed and routinely communicated with all those carers and professionals involved in a patient's care.[116]

Clinical and legal frameworks to support ACP structures are available in many countries.[117-19] In the UK, depending on jurisdiction, such guidance can cover advance statements of wishes and preferences, advance decisions to refuse treatment and the appointment of proxy decision makers. All have to be made when a patient has mental capacity to make such decisions, and they come into effect only when the patient's capacity becomes impaired.[120]

Much has been written about advance directives / decisions to refuse treatment, but, with the exception of DNACPR orders, they are rarely used. First, few people complete them.[31] Second, to be valid, the doctor needs to be sure that these were the wishes of this particular patient, the patient was competent to make this particular decision at the time of writing the directive, the directive refers specifically to the decision in question and there is no evidence of the patient having changed their mind in the interim or having been subject to coercion. Such evidence may not be available, particularly if a patient is admitted as an emergency, and specific situations can rarely be predicted in sufficient detail to cover the reality at hand.

However, the concept of considering preferences for future care and conveying these to carers and professionals, as well as family and friends, is an important principle in palliative care. Discussion and recording of wishes both for and against likely treatment modalities, in the context of individual beliefs and values, is a key part of palliative care assessment. It is a valuable tool for enhancing communication within a group of patients for who competence for decision-making may decline with increasing frailty and disease progression. Such conversations usually take place during everyday clinical care. Knowledge of patients' values and beliefs also guide best-interest decisions when unforeseen events occur.

FUTURE STRATEGIES IN HEART FAILURE PRACTICE: GENERAL ADVICE AND SPECIFIC SITUATIONS
General advice
The difficulties encountered in caring for patients with heart failure and their families have been explored. Good communications skills benefit patients, carers and professionals, and need not have a negative impact on time management. In practical terms, how can those involved in the management of heart failure patients adapt and improve their practice to address the concerns that have been discussed?

> I was told all the way through what was going to happen and why. And I think it's very important for people that one knows exactly what is going on.
>
> Female cardiac patient (Kennelly and Bowling[109])

Warmth and empathy in communication are always appreciated. However, patient expectations of the professional–patient relationship differ, and these need to be identified and negotiated.

> Communication is not just about breaking bad news . . . it is much more. Communication is about relationship – the relationships we establish and build with our patients that make the other elements of eliciting and imparting information possible.
>
> Tiernan[121]

There are a number of strategies that are best avoided:[75]

- the 'velvet-covered hand-grenade' approach, which uses jargon to avoid open discussion of the real problem and to disguise bad news, can cause confusion and resentment
- the 'hit-and-run' tactic, whereby information is given to a patient without opportunity for discussion, leaves no room for negotiation
- the 'give-it-straight' approach in response to a question can also be harmful, as it is better to explore why the patient has asked the question and to discover what they want to know before responding.

Further, it can also be difficult to judge when it is best to initiate conversations about specific concerns, such as end-of-life care or stopping treatment. Transition points have been mentioned, and, in heart failure, these are often when the patient's disease progresses from one 'stage' – for instance, NYHA class II – to the next. Another useful tactic might be for the professional to consider the question 'Would I be surprised if this patient died within the next 6 to 12 months?' – although one study using this in conjunction with other clinical indicators of poor prognosis did not demonstrate any useful correlation with survival.[122] Irrespective of estimated prognosis, a comprehensive assessment, covering the physical, psychosocial, quality-of-life and spiritual domains, would be appropriate at key transition points in the patient's illness. This could be carried out by any of the professionals involved with a patient, but decisions regarding the direction of future care are usually agreed between the patient and their doctor. Concerns, wishes and goals identified in such an assessment can lead to discussion about end-of-life care in general, and incorporate specific management decisions, such as resuscitation status, advance directives and withdrawal of medical treatment. At these points, the introduction of the concept of palliative care can be appropriate. The important point to remember, again, is that communication is a *process*, not a single event. Key points to consider are summarised in Box 7.1.

Specific situations
Breaking bad news

Breaking bad news can be one of the most challenging tasks faced by healthcare professionals.

> Bad news can be defined as any information that drastically alters a patient's view of their future for the worse.
>
> Kaye[75]

BOX 7.1 Key points to consider when communicating important issues (adapted from Kaye[76])

- Encourage the patient to bring their carer if wished.
- Ensure sufficient time and privacy if at all possible.
- Make sure you know the facts.
- Give the patient warning that the discussion is important.
- Establish what the patient already knows.
- Be open and honest.
- Explain further if the patient wishes.
- Listen to concerns and allow the expression of emotion.
- Involve patient and carer in decision-making.
- Maintain hope whenever possible.
- Avoid premature or unrealistic reassurance.
- It is always possible to offer the patient something: symptom control, psychological support or practical help.
- Summarise the discussion.
- Provide a point of contact – for example, the nurse specialist.

If done well, breaking bad news can strengthen the relationship between patient and professional and contribute positively to the partnership of managing their disease. Sometimes patients cannot understand what they have been told, use denial as a protective mechanism or become angry with the professional.[123] Such anger may also be directed at themselves, at God, or cause them to question the 'fairness' of life.

To communicate bad news is important to maintain trust and reduce uncertainty for the patient, to prevent inappropriate hope regarding their disease, to allow them time to adjust to their changing condition and to prevent a conspiracy of silence regarding their health.[75]

Prognosis

Prognostication is difficult and understudied[10] as well as being unpredictable (*see* Chapter 4, 'Prognosis in advanced heart failure'). A patient's belief that they are approaching the end of their life is strongly associated with the desire to discuss prognosis,[42] and avoiding such discussions serves only to increase the patient's distress.[124] Delay in raising the subject of prognosis can delay the diagnosis of dying, and the patient is denied the opportunity to recognise that the end of their life is approaching.[47]

As a result of a failure to prognosticate, let alone prognosticate accurately, patients may die deaths they deplore in locations they despise. They may seek noxious chemotherapy rather than good palliative care, enroll in clinical trials of experimental therapy that offer more benefit to researchers than to themselves, or reassure loved ones that it is not yet time to pay a visit – only to lapse into a coma before having a chance to say good-bye.

Christakis[125]

Many patients are unable or unwilling to consider the future when they are well and relatively symptom-free. The subject is often raised during periods of decompensation, when patients are acutely unwell. The relevance of prognosis may diminish when patients respond to medical interventions and their conditions improve. A suggested conversation between the doctor and patient may look like this:

> We know that half of people with heart failure like yours will die in the next year. We will work together to try to help you become one of the people that lives longer than that.

Pantilat and Steimle[38]

Prognosis is best presented to patients as a 'range estimate . . . with caveats',[38] given the degree of uncertainty involved. Professionals should present the situation clearly and simply, outlining the stage in their illness the patient has reached, with some communication of risk, using simple statistics if possible. Options for treatment, care and palliation of symptoms should be included in such discussions. As prognosis becomes shorter, it may be useful to use such terms as 'weeks to months', 'days to weeks' or 'hours to days'[38] to clearly convey the patient's situation to them and their family.

ICDs

ICDs are used in heart failure in an attempt to prevent premature death due to arrhythmia. Their use may also prolong the dying process and make it more distressing.[126] Once such a device is inserted, discussion regarding its deactivation can be difficult as the patient's condition progresses and the end of life approaches. Goldstein et al. noted that only 27% of carers reported that professionals had discussed deactivating ICDs.[126] Guidelines for discussing ICDs with patients and their families have been produced.[127] The majority of patients in one study recognised that such discussions are appropriate at the end of life, although a significant minority did not want their physicians to raise the subject.[8] The implications of both inserting and deactivating the device, together with consideration of advantages and disadvantages, should be discussed prior to its insertion. Specifically, the situation of the patient's overall condition having deteriorated should be discussed, including the burden the ICD may then represent.

CPR

The opinions and wishes of patients regarding resuscitation are not always sought,[47] patients often have a lack of understanding about CPR[36] and the decision to not attempt resuscitation is made on their behalf by professionals. This decision is not always communicated to the patient or their family.[128]

Guidance has been issued from many medical representative and regulatory organisations to assist professionals in making decisions regarding CPR.[129,130] As with prognosis, the timing of such a discussion can vary, but the inclusion of patients and carers can act as a catalyst for discussion of future care. However, it has been shown that patients' views on whether to agree to CPR are influenced by realistic assessments about the probability of their survival.[131]

Discussions about CPR often take place between professionals and the patient's family, as the patient may be too unwell to participate. For family members to act as surrogate decision makers and reach an informed decision, they have to be provided with all the relevant information. Approaching the subject with concern and sensitivity can reduce distress for professional, patient and carer. Communication of the patient's condition, their estimated prognosis and the predicted success of resuscitation, together with its associated negative aspects, is important. Even when well informed, relatives can feel that they are imposing a 'death sentence' on their relative by agreeing to a DNACPR order, so reassurance must be given that this is not the case.

Palliative care

Palliative care has been mentioned throughout this chapter. Often, when patients are referred to palliative care services, discussions regarding the future direction of care have already taken place. This process of communication can continue with the involvement of palliative care specialists, whose role it is to support and facilitate the patient's care and to share care with heart failure specialists and/or general practitioners.

Death and dying

The reality of *living* with advanced heart failure can mean that thoughts of approaching death may not be considered by the patient.[10] Patients can believe that professionals are reluctant to talk about death and dying, but structured and coordinated end-of-life care should be available to all patients, not just those with cancer. Care of the dying is discussed in more detail in Chapter 8, 'Care of the patient dying from heart failure'.

[I]t's this sort of roller coaster type of thing and it's very difficult to give a prognosis other than 'well it's his heart, it is serious you know'.

General practitioner (Hanratty *et al.*[84])

But even when you're at the very end and it's the last few weeks, you still don't know whether they're going to just die suddenly now or whether over the next few weeks they're just going to gradually drift away. So that does make it difficult in trying to prepare them and their relatives for what's actually going to happen.'

Cardiologist (Hanratty *et al.*[84])

SUMMARY

Good communication in palliative care and end-of-life decision-making takes time, effort and humility. It is not an easy enterprise, and the learning curve can last a lifetime. However, the rewards for effort spent are great, for patients, professionals and carers. Done well, communication at this stage of life can have a profound effect on the quality of remaining life and the death of the patient, and for the bereavement experience and memories of those dear to them. Strides have been made in professional–patient communication in general practice and oncology. Learning from patients with heart failure similarly promises to be the way forward for cardiology. If balancing and monitoring are the key aspects of physical care, then pacing and tailoring at transition points have the potential to advance communication in heart failure.

REFERENCES

1 Dias L, Chabner BA, Lynch TJ, Jr et al. Breaking bad news: a patient's perspective. *Oncologist.* 2003; 8(6): 587–96.

2 Goldacre MJ, Mant D, Duncan M et al. Mortality from heart failure in an English population, 1979–2003: study of death certification. *J Epidemiol Community Health.* 2005; 59(9): 782–4.

3 Schaufelberger M, Swedberg K, Köster M et al. Decreasing one-year mortality and hospitalization rates for heart failure in Sweden; data from the Swedish Hospital Discharge Registry 1988 to 2000. *Eur Heart J.* 2004; 25(4): 300–7.

4 Addington-Hall JM, McCarthy M. Regional Study of Care for the Dying: methods and sample characteristics. *Palliat Med.* 1995; 9(1): 27–35.

5 Murray SA, Boyd K, Kendall M et al. Dying of lung cancer or cardiac failure: prospective qualitative interview study of patients and their carers in the community. *BMJ.* 2002; 325(7370): 929.

6 Gott M, Small N, Barnes S et al. Older people's views of a good death in heart failure: implications for palliative care provision. *Soc Sci Med.* 2008; 67(7): 1113–21.

7 Barclay S, Momen N, Case-Upton S et al. End-of-life conversations with heart failure patients: a systematic literature review and narrative synthesis. *Br J Gen Pract.* 2011; 61(582): e49–62.

8 Thylén I, Moser DK, Chung ML et al. Are ICD recipients able to foresee if they want to withdraw therapy or deactivate defibrillator shocks? *Int J Cardiol Heart Vessels.* 2013; 1: 22–31.

9 McCarthy M, Lay M, Addington-Hall J. Dying from heart disease. *J R Coll Physicians Lond.* 1996; 30(4): 325–8.

10 Willems DL, Hak A, Visser F et al. Thoughts of patients with advanced heart failure on dying. *Palliat Med.* 2004; 18(6): 564–72.

11 Rogers AE, Addington-Hall JM, Abery AJ et al. Knowledge and communication difficulties for patients with chronic heart failure: qualitative study. *BMJ.* 2000; 321(7261): 605–7.

12 Rogers A, Addington-Hall JM, McCoy AS et al. A qualitative study of chronic heart failure patients' understanding of their symptoms and drug therapy. *Eur J Heart Fail.* 2002; 4(3): 283–7.

13 Caldwell PH, Arthur HM, Demers C. Preferences of patients with heart failure for prognosis communication. *Can J Cardiol.* 2007; **23**(10): 791–6.

14 Harding R, Selman L, Benyon T *et al.* Meeting the communication and information needs of chronic heart failure patients. *J Pain Symptom Manage.* 2008; **36**(2): 149–56.

15 National Institute for Health and Clinical Excellence. *Chronic Heart Failure: management of chronic heart failure in adults in primary and secondary care.* NICE guideline CG108. London: National Institute for Health and Clinical Excellence; 2010. www.nice.org.uk/guidance/CG108

16 Lang F, Floyd MR, Beine KL. Clues to patients' explanations and concerns about their illnesses. A call for active listening. *Arch Fam Med.* 2000; **9**(3): 222–7.

17 Meredith C, Symonds P, Webster L *et al.* Information needs of cancer patients in west Scotland: cross sectional survey of patients' views. *BMJ.* 1996; **313**(7059): 724–6.

18 Holman H, Lorig K. Patients as partners in managing chronic disease. Partnership is a prerequisite for effective and efficient health care. *BMJ.* 2000; **320**(7234): 526–7.

19 Fallowfield L, Jenkins V, Farewell V *et al.* Efficacy of a Cancer Research UK communication skills training model for oncologists: a randomised controlled trial. *Lancet.* 2002; **359**(9307): 650–6.

20 Hope CJ, Wu, J, Tu W *et al.* Association of medication adherence, knowledge, and skills with emergency department visits by adults 50 years or older with congestive heart failure. *Am J Health Syst Pharm.* 2004; **61**(19): 2043–9.

21 Moser DK, Dracup K. Psychosocial recovery from a cardiac event: the influence of perceived control. *Heart Lung.* 1995; **24**(4): 273–80.

22 Edmonds P, Rogers A. 'If only someone had told me . . .' A review of the care of patients dying in hospital. *Clin Med.* 2003; **3**(2): 149–52.

23 Ahluwalia SC, Levin JR, Lorenz KA *et al.* Missed opportunities for advance care planning communication during outpatient clinic visits. *J Gen Intern Med.* 2011; **27**(4): 445–51.

24 Artinian NT, Magnan M, Christian W *et al.* What do patients know about their heart failure? *Appl Nurs Res.* 2002; **15**(4): 200–8.

25 Chan AD, Reid GJ, Farvolden P *et al.* Learning needs of patients with congestive heart failure. *Can J Cardiol.* 2003; **19**(4): 413–17.

26 Koelling TM, Johnson ML, Cody RJ *et al.* Discharge education improves clinical outcomes in patients with chronic heart failure. *Circulation.* 2005; **111**(2): 179–85.

27 Barnes S, Gott M, Payne S *et al.* Communication in heart failure: perspectives from older people and primary care professionals. *Health Soc Care Comm.* 2006; **14**(6): 482–90.

28 Selman L, Harding R, Benyon T *et al.* Improving end-of-life care for patients with chronic heart failure: 'Let's hope it'll get better, when I know in my heart of hearts it won't'. *Heart.* 2007; **93**(8): 963–7.

29 Beng KS. The last hours and days of life: a biopsychosocial–spiritual model of care. *Asia Pac Fam Med.* 2004; **4**: 1–3.

30 Hopper SV, Fischback RL. Patient-physician communication when blindness threatens. *Patient Educ Couns.* 1989; **14**(1): 69–79.

31 Formiga F, Chivite D, Ortega C *et al.* End-of-life preferences in elderly patients admitted for heart failure. *QJM.* 2004; **97**(12): 803–8.

32 McCarthy M, Addington-Hall J, Ley M. Communication and choice in dying from heart disease. *J R Soc Med.* 1997; **90**(3): 128–31.

33 Wotton K, Borbasi S, Redden M. When all else has failed: nurses' perception of factors influencing palliative care for patients with end-stage heart failure. *J Cardiovasc Nurs.* 2005; **20**(1): 18–25.

34 Boyd KJ, Murray SA, Kendall M *et al.* Living with advanced heart failure: a prospective, community based study of patients and their carers. *Eur J Heart Fail.* 2004; **6**(5): 585–91.

35 Löfmark R, Nilstun T. Not if, but how: one way to talk with patients about forgoing life support. *Postgrad Med J.* 2000; **76**(891): 26–8.

36 Strachan PH, Ross H, Rocker GM *et al.* Mind the gap: opportunities for improving end-of-life care for patients with advanced heart failure. *Can J Cardiol.* 2009; **25**(11): 635–40.

37 Gibbs LM, Addington-Hall J, Gibbs JS. Dying from heart failure: lessons from palliative care. Many patients would benefit from palliative care at the end of their lives. *BMJ.* 1998; **317**(7164): 961–2.

38 Pantilat SZ, Steimle AE. Palliative care for patients with heart failure. *JAMA.* 2004; **291**(20): 2476–82.

39 Stewart K. Discussing cardiopulmonary resuscitation with patients and relatives. *Postgrad Med J.* 1995; **71**(840): 585–9.

40 Mackillop WJ, Stewart WE, Ginsburg AD *et al.* Cancer patients' perceptions of their disease and its treatment. *Br J Cancer.* 1988; **58**(3): 355–8.

41 Weeks JC, Cook EF, O'Day SJ *et al.* Relationship between cancer patients' predictions of prognosis and their treatment preferences. *JAMA.* 1998; **279**(21): 1709–14.

42 Fried TR, Bradley EH, O'Leary J. Prognosis communication in serious illness: perceptions of older patients, caregivers, and clinicians. *J Am Ger Soc.* 2003; **51**(10): 1398–403.

43 Kutner JS, Steiner JF, Corbett KK *et al.* Information needs in terminal illness. *Soc Sci Med.* 1999; **48**(10): 1341–52.

44 Leydon GM, Boulton M, Moynihan C *et al.* Cancer patients' information needs and information seeking behaviour: in depth interview study. *BMJ.* 2000; **320**(7239): 909–13.

45 Murray SA, Boyd K, Sheikh A. Palliative care in chronic illness. *BMJ.* 2005; **330**(7498): 611–12.

46 Dudley N. Importance of risk communication and decision making in cardiovascular conditions in older patients: a discussion paper. *Qual Health Care.* 2001; **10**(Suppl. 1): i19–22.

47 Gibbs JS. Heart disease. In: Addington-Hall JM, Higginson IJ, editors. *Palliative Care for Non-Cancer Patients.* Oxford: Oxford University Press; 2005. pp. 30–43.

48 Wenger NK. Quality of life: can it and should it be assessed in patients with heart failure? *Cardiology.* 1989; **76**(5): 391–8.

49 Freedland KE, Carney RM, Rich MW *et al.* Depression in elderly patients with congestive heart failure. *J Geriatr Psychiatry.* 1991; **24**: 59–71.

50 Koenig HG. Depression in hospitalized older patients with congestive heart failure. *Gen Hosp Psychiatry.* 1998; **20**(1): 29–43.

51 Frasure-Smith N, Lespérance F, Talajic M. Depression following myocardial infarction. Impact on 6-month survival. *JAMA.* 1993; **270**(15): 1819–25.

52 Rabins PV, Harvis K, Koven S. High fatality rates of late-life depression associated with cardiovascular disease. *J Affect Disord.* 1985; 9(2): 165–7.

53 Carney RM, Rich MW, Freedland KE *et al.* Major depressive disorder predicts cardiac events in patients with coronary artery disease. *Psychosom Med.* 1988; 50(6): 627–33.

54 Carney RM, Freedland KE, Eisen SA *et al.* Major depression and medication adherence in elderly patients with coronary artery disease. *Health Psychol.* 1995; 14(1): 88–90.

55 Dunbar J. Predictors of patient adherence: patient characteristics. In: Shumaker SA, Schron EB, Ockene JK, editors. *The Handbook of Health Behaviour Change.* New York, NY: Springer; 1998. pp. 348–60.

56 Hawthorne MH, Hixon ME. Functional status, mood disturbance and quality of life in patients with heart failure. *Prog Cardiovasc Nursing.* 1994; 9(1): 22–32.

57 Maricle RA, Hosenpud JD, Norman DJ *et al.* Depression in patients being evaluated for heart transplantation. *Gen Hosp Psychiatry.* 1989; 11(6): 418–24.

58 Tung EE, North F. Advance care planning in the primary care setting: a comparison of attending staff and resident barriers. *Am J Hosp Palliat Care.* 2009; 26(6): 456–63.

59 Ramsaroop SD, Reid MC, Adelman RD. Completing an advance directive in the primary care setting: what do we need for success? *J Am Geriatr Soc.* 2007; 55(2): 277–83.

60 Costello J. Truth telling and the dying patient: a conspiracy of silence? *Int J Palliat Nurs.* 2000; 6(8): 398–405.

61 Wehby D, Brenner PS. Perceived learning needs of patients with heart failure. *Heart Lung.* 1999; 28(1): 31–40.

62 Gott M, Barnes S, Parker C *et al.* Dying trajectories in heart failure. *Palliat Med.* 2007; 21(2): 95–9.

63 Franciosa JA, Wilen M, Ziesche S *et al.* Survival in men with severe chronic left ventricular failure due to either coronary heart disease or idiopathic dilated cardiomyopathy. *Am J Cardiol.* 1983; 51(5): 831–6.

64 Gradman A, Deedwania P, Cody R *et al.* Predictors of total mortality and sudden death in mild to moderate heart failure. Captopril-Digoxin Study Group. *J Am Coll Cardiol.* 1989; 14(3): 564–70; discussion 571–2.

65 Kjekshus J. Arrhythmias and mortality in congestive heart failure. *Am J Cardiol.* 1990; 65(19): 42–8.

66 Cooperative North Scandinavian Enalapril Survival Study (CONSENSUS) Trial Study Group. Effects of enalapril on mortality in severe congestive heart failure. Results of the Cooperative North Scandinavian Enalapril Survival Study (CONSENSUS). *N Engl J Med.* 1997; 316(23): 1429–35.

67 Tayler M, Ogden J. Doctors' use of euphemisms and their impact on patients' beliefs about health: an experimental study of heart failure. *Patient Educ Couns.* 2005; 57(3): 321–6.

68 Christakis NA, Iwashyna TJ. Attitude and self-reported practice regarding prognostication in a national sample of internists. *Arch Int Med.* 1998; 158(21): 2389–95.

69 Lamont EB, Christakis NA. Complexities in prognostication in advanced cancer: 'to help them live their lives the way they want to'. *JAMA.* 2003; 290(1): 98–104.

70 Kurtz S, Silverman J, Draper J. *Teaching and Learning Communication Skills in Medicine.* 2nd ed. Abingdon, Oxon: Radcliffe Medical Press; 2005.

71 Silverman J, Kurtz S, Draper J. *Skills for Communicating with Patients.* 2nd ed. Abingdon, Oxon: Radcliffe Medical Press; 2005.

72 Makoul G. Communication skills education in medical school and beyond. *JAMA.* 2003; **289**(1): 93.

73 Emanuel EJ, Emanuel LL. Four models of the physician-patient relationship. *JAMA.* 1992; **267**(16): 2221–6.

74 Randall F, Downie RS. *Palliative Care Ethics: a companion for all specialties.* 2nd ed. Oxford: Oxford University Press; 1999.

75 Kaye P. *Breaking Bad News: a 10 step approach.* Northampton: EPL; 1996.

76 Bradley RH, Cramer LD, Bogardus ST, Jr *et al.* Physicians' ratings of their knowledge, attitudes, and end-of-life practices. *Acad Med.* 2002; **77**(4): 305–11.

77 Beattie J, Connolly M. Managing the end-game: palliative care for advanced heart failure. *Heart Improvement eBulletin.* 2009; **April/May:** 11–12. Available at: http://system. improvement.nhs.uk/ImprovementSystem/ViewDocument.aspx?path=Cardiac/ National/Website/Heart/managing%20the%20end%20game%20article.pdf (accessed 16 April 2014)

78 Statham H, Dimavicius J. Commentary: how do you give the bad news to parents? *Birth.* 1992; **19**(2): 103–4.

79 Buckman R. Breaking bad news: why is it still so difficult? *Br Med J (Clin Res Ed).* 1984; **288**(6430): 1597–9.

80 Speck P. Communication skills. Breaking bad news. *Nurs Times.* 1991; **87**(12): 24–6.

81 Maguire P, Pitceathley C. Key communication skills and how to acquire them. *BMJ.* 2002; **325**(7366): 697–700.

82 Apatira L, Boyd EA, Malvar G *et al.* Hope, truth, and preparing for death: perspectives of surrogate decision makers. *Ann Intern Med.* 2008; **149**(12): 861–8.

83 Clayton JM, Hancock K, Parker S *et al.* Sustaining hope when communicating with terminally ill patients and their families: a systematic review. *Psychooncology.* 2008; **17**(7): 641–59.

84 Hanratty B, Hibbert D, Mair F *et al.* Doctors' perceptions of palliative care for heart failure: focus group study. *BMJ.* 2002; **325**(7364): 581–5.

85 Oken D. What to tell cancer patients. A study of medical attitudes. *JAMA.* 1961; **175**: 1120–8.

86 Charlton RC. Breaking bad news. *Med J Aust.* 1992; **157**(9): 615–21.

87 Goldberg RJ. Disclosure of information to adult cancer patients: issues and update. *J Clin Oncol.* 1984; **2**(8): 948–55.

88 Woodward LJ, Pamies RL. The disclosure of the diagnosis of cancer. *Prim Care.* 1992; **19**(4): 657–63.

89 National Institute for Clinical Excellence. *Improving Supportive and Palliative Care for Adults with Cancer: the manual.* London: National Institute for Clinical Excellence; 2004. Available at: www.nice.org.uk/guidance/csgsp/resources/supportive-and-palliative-care-the-manual-2 (accessed 22 May 2015).

90 Fallowfield LJ, Jenkins VA, Beveridge HA. Truth may hurt but deceit hurts more: communication in palliative care. *Palliat Med.* 2002; **16**(4): 297–303.

91 Fallowfield L, Saul J, Gilligan B. Teaching senior nurses how to teach communication skills in oncology. *Cancer Nurs.* 2001; **24**(3): 185–91.

92 Razavi D, Delvaux N, Marchal S *et al.* The effects of a 24-h psychological training

program on attitudes, communication skills and occupational stress in oncology: a randomised study. *Eur J Cancer.* 1993; **29**(13): 1858–63.

93 Wilkinson S, Bailey K, Aldridge J et al. A longitudinal evaluation of a communication skills programme. *Palliat Med.* 1999; **13**(4): 341–8.

94 Buckman R. *How to Break Bad News: a guide for health care professionals.* London: Papermac; 1994.

95 Parle M, Jones B, Maguire P. Maladaptive coping and affective disorders among cancer patients. *Psychol Med.* 1996; **26**(4): 735–44.

96 Heaven CM, Maguire P. Disclosure of concerns by hospice patients and their identification by nurses. *Palliat Med.* 1997; **11**(4): 283–90.

97 Fellowes D, Wilkinson S, Moore P. Communication skills training for health care professionals working with cancer patients, their families and/or carers. *Cochrane Database Syst Rev.* 2004; (2): CD003751.

98 Aspegren K. BEME Guide No. 2: Teaching and learning communication skills in medicine-a review with quality grading of articles. *Med Teach.* 1999; **21**(6): 563–70.

99 Maguire P, Booth K, Elliott C et al. Helping health professionals involved in cancer care acquire key interviewing skills – the impact of workshops. *Eur J Cancer.* 1996; **32A**(9): 1486–9.

100 Krumholz HM, Amatruda J, Smith GL et al. Randomized trial of an education and support intervention to prevent readmission of patients with heart failure. *J Am Coll Cardiol.* 2002; **39**(1): 83–9.

101 Strömberg A. Educating nurses and patients to manage heart failure. *Eur J Cardiovasc Nurs.* 2002; **1**(1): 33–40.

102 Ogden J, Branson R, Bryett A et al. What's in a name? An experimental study of patients' views of the impact and function of a diagnosis. *Fam Pract.* 2003; **20**(3): 248–53.

103 Horne G, Payne S. Removing the boundaries: palliative care for patients with heart failure. *Palliat Med.* 2004; **18**(4): 291–6.

104 Skolones LC. The meaning of heart failure. *Crit Care Nurs.* 2008; **28**(4): 17–18; author reply 18.

105 Zambroski CH. Qualitative analysis of living with heart failure. *Heart Lung.* 2003; **32**(1): 32–40.

106 Edmonds PM, Rogers A, Addington-Hall JM et al. Patient descriptors of breathlessness in heart failure. *Int J Cardiol.* 2005; **98**(1): 61–6.

107 Green E, Gardiner C, Gott M et al. Exploring the extent of communication surrounding transitions to palliative care in heart failure: the perspectives of health care professionals. *J Palliat Care.* 2011; **27**(2): 107–16.

108 Sayers GM, Barratt D, Gothard C et al. The value of taking an 'ethics history'. *J Med Eth.* 2001; **27**(2): 114–7.

109 Kennelly C, Bowling A. Suffering in deference: a focus group study of older cardiac patients' preferences for treatment and perceptions of risk. *Qual Health Care.* 2001; **10**(Suppl. 1): i23–8.

110 Heart and Stroke Foundation of Ontario. *End of Life Planning and Care for Heart Failure Patients: summary for the Heart Failure End-of-Life Planning and Care Task Group.* Toronto, ON: Heart and Stroke Foundation of Ontario; 2010. Available at: www. heartandstroke.on.ca/atf/cf/%7B33c6fa68-b56b-4760-abc6-d85b2d02ee71%7D/

END%20OF%20LIFE%20PLANNING%20AND%20CARE%20FOR%20HF%20 PATIENTSF.PDF (accessed 22 May 2015).

111 Connolly M, Beattie J, Walker D *et al. End of Life Care in Heart Failure: a framework for implementation.* London: National End of Life Care Programme; 2010. Available at: improvementsystem.nhsiq.nhs.uk/ImprovementSystem/ViewDocument. aspx?path=Cardiac/National/Website/Heart/Heart Failure/EOL_in_HF.pdf (accessed 22 May 2015).

112 Heart Failure Society of America. HFSA 2010 comprehensive heart failure practice guideline. *J Card Fail.* 2010; **16**(6): e1–2.

113 NHS National End of Life Care Programme. *Capacity, Care Planning and Advance Care Planning in Life Limiting Illness.* Leicester: NHS National End of Life Care Programme; 2011. Available at: www.ncpc.org.uk/sites/default/files/ACP_Booklet_June_2011.pdf (accessed 17 April 2014).

114 Schonfeld TL, Stevens EA, Lampman MM *et al.* Assessing challenges in end-of-life conversations with elderly patients with multiple morbidities. *Am J Hosp Palliat Care.* 2010; **29**(4): 260–7.

115 Johnson M, Nunn A, Hawkes T *et al.* Planning for end-of-life care in heart failure: experience of two integrated cardiology-palliative care teams. *Br J Cardiol.* 2010; **19**(2): 71–5.

116 Scottish Partnership for Palliative Care. *Living and Dying with Advanced Heart Failure: a palliative care approach.* Edinburgh: Scottish Partnership for Palliative Care; 2008. Available at: www.palliativecarescotland.org.uk/content/publications/HF-final-document.pdf (accessed 22 May 2015).

117 Howlett J, Morrin L, Fortin M *et al.* End-of-life planning in heart failure: it should be the end of the beginning. *Can J Cardiol.* 2010; **26**(3): 135–41.

118 Janssen DJ, Spruit MA, Schols JM *et al.* A call for high-quality advance care planning in outpatients with severe COPD or chronic heart failure. *Chest.* 2011; **139**(5): 1081–8.

119 Karver SB, Berger J. The importance of discussing living wills with patients with heart failure. *Rev Esp Cardiol.* 2010; **63**(12): 1396–8. [Article in English and Spanish.]

120 Mental Capacity Act 2005. London: HM Government; 7 April 2005. Available at: www.legislation.gov.uk/ukpga/2005/9/pdfs/ukpga_20050009_en.pdf (accessed 22 May 2015).

121 Tiernan E. Communication training for professionals. *Support Care Cancer.* 2003; **11**(12): 758–62.

122 Haga K, Murray S, Reid J *et al.* Identifying community based chronic heart failure patients in the last year of life: a comparison of the Gold Standards Framework Prognostic Indicator Guide and the Seattle Heart Failure Model. *Heart.* 2012; **98**(7): 579–83.

123 Lloyd-Williams M. Breaking bad news to patients and relatives. *BMJ.* 2002; **325**: s11–12.

124 Stedeford A. *Facing Death: patients, families and professionals.* London: Heinemann; 1984.

125 Christakis NA. *Death Foretold: prophecy and prognosis in medical care.* Chicago, IL: University of Chicago Press; 1999.

126 Goldstein NE, Lampert R, Bradley E *et al.* Management of implantable cardioverter defibrillators in end-of-life care. *Ann Intern Med.* 2004; **141**(11): 835–8.

127 Harrington MD, Luebke DL, Lewis WR *et al.* *Implantable Cardioverter-Defibrillator at End-of-Life.* Fast Fact number 112. 2004. Available at: www.capc.org/fast-facts/112-implantable-cardioverter-defibrillators-end-life/ (accessed 22 May 2015).

128 Löfmark R, Nilstun T. Do-not-resuscitate orders – should the patient be informed? *J Intern Med.* 1997; **241**(5): 421–5.

129 British Medical Association. *Withholding and Withdrawing Life-Prolonging Medical Treatment: guidance for decision making.* 2nd ed. London: BMJ Books; 2001.

130 General Medical Council (GMC). *Withholding and Withdrawing Life-prolonging Treatments: good practice in decision-making.* London: GMC; 2002.

131 Murphy DJ, Burrows D, Santilli S *et al.* The influence of the probability of survival on patients' preferences regarding cardiopulmonary resuscitation. *N Engl J Med.* 1994; **330**(8): 545–9.

132 Ellershaw J, Ward C. Care of the dying patient: the last hours or days of life. *BMJ.* 2003; **326**(7379): 30–4.

Care of the patient dying from heart failure

HILLARY LUM AND DAVID BEKELMAN

INTRODUCTION

Care of the patient dying from heart failure is an integral part of the healthcare provider's role. Optimal care for the dying patient requires close partnership between the patient, family members and healthcare team. The priority in management is the assessment of the final goals of the patient and family regarding medical, psychosocial and spiritual needs.[1]

Patients with heart failure are more likely to die of progressive heart failure than sudden death, often late in the disease course, when heart failure symptoms are severe and long-standing.[2] The modern heart failure regimen has reduced mortality from sudden cardiac death and increased the time a patient lives with heart failure. The implantable cardiovertor defibrillator (ICD) and beta-blockers have played a large part in the primary and secondary prevention of death from ventricular tachyarrhythmias. Thus, this chapter focuses on the care of the patient dying of progressive heart failure and their families.

Given the significant advances in cardiac technologies and the frequent remissions from exacerbations of heart failure, it can be challenging for patients, families and their healthcare team to shift from a disease-focused, life-prolonging care model to a care model in which the goal is to provide physical, psychological, social and spiritual care to the patient and family in the last days of life. While some needs and skills required to care for a patient dying from heart failure are similar to those required to care for a patient dying from other illnesses, this chapter focuses on specific issues that patients dying of heart failure face, including recognition of the dying phase, needs during the last days of life, the impact of advanced cardiac technologies and practical approaches to care.

GOOD DEATH: CONCEPT AND IMPORTANCE OF LOCATION

The concept of a 'good death' is critical to framing the needs and approaches to caring for the dying patient. Seriously ill patients, recently bereaved family members and healthcare team members identified important attributes of quality at the end of life, both in general and when dying from heart failure (*see* Box 8.1).[3] While many of these factors were important to most individuals, specific components of a good death should be expected to vary, based on the individual's specific values, experiences, cultural and religious background, and beliefs.

BOX 8.1 A good death

*According to patients with chronic illness, bereaved family members and healthcare providers**

- Respect for treatment preferences
- Pain and symptom management
- Preparation for death
- Achieving a sense of completion
- Being treated as a 'whole person'

*According to patients with heart failure***

- Sudden death
- Opportunity to discuss where and how death occurs
- Death at home
- Focus on comfort, including symptom relief
- Reducing emotional and physical burdens on family
- Honest communication
- Avoiding unnecessary interventions

Notes: *Adapted from Steinhauser *et al.*[3] **Adapted from Strachan *et al.*,[4] Dougherty *et al.*,[18] Hopp *et al.*,[19] Small *et al.*[22] and Murray *et al.*[52]

In the context of the patient's concept of a good death, location of the last days of life may be quite significant. Although some patients with heart failure expressed a preference to die at home,[4] among US patients with heart failure who died in 2007, 35% died in the hospital (50% of this group in the intensive-care unit), whereas 35% utilised hospice care at the time of death.[5] There are significant differences in the resources available to patient and family during the dying phase, depending on whether they are at home, have hospice services or are in the hospital. For patients who desire to die at home, healthcare providers need to work closely with family to identify tangible options for assuring good symptom control and meeting the other needs of the actively dying person. This may be helped by frameworks of care, such as the Gold Standards Framework and other community-based palliative care programmes.[6]

Hospice care is regarded as the gold standard of care for those who desire to die outside of the hospital, though it may be underutilised given patient or healthcare provider barriers to referral or referrals very close to the last days of life.[7] Hospice programmes are uniquely equipped to support the actively dying patient and their family through coordination to meet practical care needs, education and skilled communication, after-hours availability, and bereavement care. For individuals who may choose to die in the hospital, or lack support to meet their care needs outside of the hospital, inpatient palliative care consultation may improve the care of dying patients and support for family and staff, and has been associated with reduced invasive and expensive treatments.[8] If a patient's concept of a good death includes dying at home, early recognition of the dying phase is essential to help the patient and family identify resources to return home if possible and avoid future hospitalisations. An analysis of a large representative UK primary care database showed that not only were fewer patients dying from heart failure placed on a palliative care register before death than those dying from cancer (7% versus 48%), but that of those who were registered, a third were registered within a week of death: a challenging timescale within which to put sufficient community support in place.[9]

RECOGNITION OF THE DYING PHASE

Recognition of the dying phase is important, because it prompts healthcare providers to help the patient and family shift goals from life-prolonging treatment to care for the dying. The patient and family can then discuss preferences for care and psychological or spiritual experiences can be facilitated, such as reconciling with family or considering issues of meaning and purpose. In heart failure, recognition of the dying phase is challenged by several barriers, including concern that a disease exacerbation may be potentially reversible.[10] Even in its advanced stages, heart failure remains a disease of exacerbations and remissions. As discussed in Chapter 4, 'Prognosis in advanced heart failure', prognostication is very challenging. Among 1404 patients hospitalised for an acute heart failure exacerbation who actually were within 3 days of death, the median statistical model-based estimate of 6-month survival was 54%.[11] The challenge is recognising which disease exacerbation is likely to be the last deterioration.

There are no validated tools to identify patients who are dying of heart failure. Practical clinical questions that may aid in the diagnosis of dying are included in Table 8.1.[12] 'Consider Palliative Care', a screening tool adopted in some US Veterans Administration medical centres, and the 'Palliative Performance Scale' are general tools that may also help trigger recognition of the dying phase.[13,14] Ellershaw and Ward have suggested additional indicators that describe a heart failure patient who is at high risk of entering the active dying phase.[10] Table 8.1 also shows heart failure-specific and general indicators that suggest a patient may be approaching the last days of life and common signs and symptoms of the active dying phase.

TABLE 8.1 Recognising the active dying heart failure patient

Practical questions to assess for terminal care	Indicators of high risk of entering the active dying process		Common signs and symptoms of the active dying phase
	Heart failure-specific indicators	General indicators*	
• Could this patient be in the last days of life?	• Previous hospitalisations with worsening heart failure	• Confined to bed or chair and unable to perform self-care activities	• Audible retained respiratory secretions
• Was this patient's condition expected to deteriorate in this way?	• No identifiable reversible precipitant	• Increasingly drowsy or semi-comatose state	• Tachypnoea (respiratory rate >20 per minute)
• Is further life-prolonging treatment inappropriate?	• Declining functional status despite improving volume status	• Minimal fluid intake	• Sustained tachycardia at rest (HF >100 beats per minute)
• Have potentially reversible causes of deterioration been excluded?	• Inability to tolerate guideline-indicated therapy due to adverse effects or medical co-morbidities	• Inability to take oral medications	• Mottling or cyanosis of extremities
	• Deteriorating renal function	• Length of stay >7 days	• Decreasing level of consciousness
	• Failure to respond within 2–3 days to appropriate changes in diuretic or vasodilator drugs		• Decreasing pulses

Note: *A patient entering the dying phase usually has at least two of the following four general indicators: (1) bed bound, (2) semi-conscious, (3) only taking sips of fluid and (4) unable to take oral medication.

HF = heart failure.

Source: Adapted from Ellershaw and Ward,[10] Boyd and Murray[12] and Bailey et al.[13]

NEEDS OF THE PATIENT DYING FROM HEART FAILURE

There is limited research focused on the specific needs of heart failure patients who are in their final days of life. Key areas of need for the dying patient and their family include clear communication; physical, psychological, social and spiritual care needs; and caregiver needs during the dying phase and bereavement.

Communication

Communication to patients and families that the dying phase has begun provides an opportunity for the patient, their family and the healthcare team to discuss the patient's values and preferences for the final phase of life.[1] Additionally, it provides spiritual and psychological opportunities for the patient and family, such as life review and expressions of gratitude, apology or forgiveness. As described in Chapters 7 and 9, the optimal situation for patients with heart failure is for communication related to goals-of-care discussions, advance care planning and shared decision-making to be part of an ongoing process from the time of diagnosis. As indicators of the active dying phase are observed, the healthcare team should be in agreement that the patient is entering the final phase of life to enable discussions with the patient and family about final needs and wishes. Communication related to the dying process should include eliciting or revisiting the individual's concept of a good death; preferences for location of care leading up to death; role of current cardiac therapies and resuscitation attempts; and practical needs, such as the availability of caregivers, support and community resources (Table 8.2). As the patient enters the active dying phase, the healthcare team will often be communicating with family members, as cognitive impairment in patients dying of heart failure is common.[15] Later in this chapter, we discuss specific issues related to discussing the withdrawal of advanced cardiac therapies, such as ICDs or left ventricular assist devices (LVADs).

Physical needs

Patients with progressive heart failure have a significant symptom burden, as described in Chapter 5, 'Symptom relief for advanced heart failure'. The active dying phase may include a worsening of symptoms or development of new symptoms that require an escalation in management to relieve suffering. At the time of admission to home-hospice services, a cohort of 40 patients with heart failure reported experiencing an average of 12 symptoms (range, 0–32), with the most prevalent symptoms being dry mouth (72.5%), lack of energy (70%) and shortness of breath (65%).[16] In the last week of life, documented symptoms in 90 patients receiving hospice care included shortness of breath (60%), oedema (43%), incontinence of bowel and/or bladder (37%) and confusion at least some of the time (48%).[17] The number and severity of symptoms are frequently influenced by the presence of multiple medical conditions. Older, frail patients with heart failure often have medical co-morbidities such as chronic kidney disease, anaemia, respiratory disease and dementia, as well as problems

TABLE 8.2 Practical communication skills and sample language for care during the dying phase

Communication skill	Aspect(s) of communication	Sample phrase(s)
Establish the setting and participants	Determine who should be present, including appropriate healthcare team members or family that the patient would like to be aware of the dying phase	'For our meeting, I'm going to have [a hospice representative] be part of our conversation. In terms of your family or support network, who would you like to be here?'
Determine what patient/family know and want to know	Ask what patient/family knows	'What is your sense of what is occurring now?'
	Ask what patient/family want to know	'How much information would you like about what is happening now?'
Discuss difficult news	Tell the patient/family that the patient is dying in a sympathetic, thoughtful and clear manner	'While I hoped we could reverse your situation, I am concerned you are dying from heart failure.'
	Ask the patient/family to respond to assess understanding and provide support	'Can you tell me more about what you're thinking right now?'
Establish goals and preferences	Use open-ended questions to learn about the patient's values and what is important for a good death	'What is important to you now?' 'What are you hoping for?' 'What are some of your concerns?'
Work with patient/family to tailor care to patient goals	Discuss risks/benefits/burdens of particular therapies (i.e. resuscitation, medications, advanced cardiac technologies)	'At this point, [medical intervention] is no longer providing you with benefit. I recommend that we focus on treatments that lead to comfort and stop [medical intervention].'
	Identify practical considerations for end-of-life care (i.e. location of care, preferred healthcare team, availability of caregivers)	'If you choose to go home, which family or friends are available to help out? How much care can they realistically support at home?' 'Based on what you've told me of your needs, I'd recommend hospice to provide more support at home. Can we talk about that?'
Discuss the dying process	Tailor information to what patient/family want to know	'There are a few aspects of the dying process we can discuss. How much detail would you like to know about what is happening and how we will work for your comfort?'

Source: Adapted from Allen *et al.*[26] and Hansen-Flaschen.[53]

common in the elderly such as falls, delirium, cognitive impairment and urinary incontinence.[15] For many patients, reduced cardiac output and poor oral intake as they enter the active dying phase will drive renal dysfunction, with resulting lethargy, nausea, poor appetite and delirium. A comprehensive symptom assessment with a patient-centred approach and attention to multiple medical conditions is recommended to determine which interventions are likely to improve symptom burden and which therapies are no longer appropriate as the patient enters the last days of life.

Psychological, social and spiritual needs

Leading up to the last days of life, patients may experience changes in their psychological, social and spiritual levels of distress. First-person accounts from patients with heart failure frequently describe thinking and talking about death, including where and how they may die as a result of their heart failure.[18] Some patients retrospectively examine their lives and feel a sense of contentment in the final phase of life, while others want to hasten death.[19] Sometimes, patients have fewer needs in these domains during the dying phase, as many are extremely fatigued, have decreased levels of wakefulness or have progressive cognitive impairment. Some develop confusional states (delirium) and management of agitated behaviours is required.

Caregiver needs

Heart failure patients and caregivers have distinct needs related to the unique trajectory of heart failure with its high levels of uncertainty, including frequent periods of disease exacerbation.[20,21] Information is needed to understand and support the specific needs of caregivers of patients with heart failure during the last days of life. Qualitative interviews with bereaved caregivers captured reflections on the time of death itself; in particular, caregivers noted its suddenness and the medical care that was available when it occurred, including how hospital and home deaths were experienced in different ways.[22] When death occurred in the hospital, several caregivers felt that there were too many unnecessary interventions.[22]

Caregivers of patients with heart failure also have bereavement needs related to grief and distress after the patient dies. Caregivers reported adopting a range of coping strategies to deal with grief including 'using their faith' and 'busying themselves' with practicalities.[22] While most caregivers reported receiving no specific bereavement support, some felt that professional input would be helpful. There was satisfaction with services accessed during the bereavement period, although only a small number engaged in bereavement counselling.[22] The caregiver perspective highlighted that the concept of a good death includes both patient choice and caregiver needs. Given that caregivers are part of the social context in which death occurs, the healthcare team should recognise that the individual's death does not stop the need to plan for the ongoing care and support of caregivers.

ADVANCED TECHNOLOGIES IN THE DYING PHASE

As described in Chapter 3, 'Optimal therapy for heart failure', a number of people with advanced heart failure will be treated with advanced technologies, including ICDs, cardiac resynchronisation and LVADs. For some patients who are living with advanced disease or even in the last days of life, the potential availability of these therapies will affect decision-making about whether the technology can potentially benefit them or whether a transition to comfort-oriented care is appropriate given their goals and preferences. It is important to recognise whether the patient is likely to be in the dying phase, irrespective of available treatments, since aggressive procedures in the final days of life (including intubation and ICD implantation in patients who are not anticipated to experience clinical improvement) are not appropriate.[23] This section focuses on specific considerations for the dying patient when an advanced cardiac technology is already in place.

The withdrawal of advanced cardiac technologies may lead to unique symptom needs related to rapid progression through the dying phase. These situations may be emotionally difficult for patients, family members and the healthcare team. Practical, case-based discussions of ethical considerations related to the withdrawal of cardiac medications and cardiac devices exist.[24,25] As physical, psychological, social and spiritual care is provided, each person involved should remember that respect for patient autonomy means healthcare team members should respect autonomous patient or authorised surrogate requests to withdraw or discontinue medical therapies, even when these therapies are life prolonging, working within relevant professional and legal frameworks.

ICDs

As ICDs perform the same function as external defibrillation, when a patient in the dying phase makes a decision to forego external resuscitation, there should be an accompanying discussion that device deactivation is an option. Current guidelines recommend discussing ICD deactivation to avoid unnecessary pain and distress for patients and families.[23,26] In a retrospective study of 130 Swedish decedents that included post-mortem ICD interrogation, 35% had a ventricular arrhythmia in the last hour before death and 31% received a shock in the last 24 hours.[27] Also in this study, 65 patients had a 'do not attempt cardiopulmonary resuscitation' order and 33 of their devices (51%) were still noted to be 'on' 1 hour prior to death. Even in the hospice setting, less than 10% of US hospice agencies had a policy regarding ICD deactivation, and more than 50% of hospices reported at least one patient who had been shocked within the past year.[28]

However, while the option of ICD deactivation should be discussed prior to the last days of life, only 27% of patients and families had discussed deactivation at any time preceding death[29] and US physicians, including cardiologists and primary care physicians, reported low rates of discussions with patients or families.[30] Demonstrating the need for discussions about ICD deactivation, a national survey of Swedish ICD recipients found that insufficient knowledge about the role of the ICD was common and associated with choosing to keep the shock therapy of the ICD even when dying from cancer or other serious chronic illnesses.[31] Nearly one-third (28%) believed that deactivation was equal to active euthanasia, and the overwhelming majority believed that reprogramming to pacing mode only would result in immediate death. Taken together, a discussion about the option of ICD deactivation will frequently become the responsibility of the healthcare team caring for the patient dying of heart failure and will require dedicated patient-centred education and counselling. Finally, some patients may choose to keep an ICD active while electing to forego external resuscitation. While this may be consistent with a patient's wishes, and in some cases appropriate (e.g. when immediate defibrillation is likely to be successful, but the patient lives at a distance from emergency services), more often it is due to misunderstandings about care goals or the meaning of ICD deactivation.[32]

Pacemakers

Patients and families may request that a pacemaker, including a biventricular pacing device, be turned off during the active dying phase.[33] The exact clinical experience after pacemaker deactivation will vary by patient. If the patient is dependent on pacemaker function, death may be hastened by turning the rate down to the minimum 30 beats per minute. Some patients may experience the reappearance of the symptoms the pacemaker was placed to alleviate. It is also possible that as death due to progressive heart failure occurs, the myocardium will become less responsive to pacemaker stimulation and pacemaker function will become irrelevant. Thus, it is hard to anticipate the effect of pacemaker deactivation on the dying process. If the patient's goal is not to prolong death by any means, providers should discuss the possibility of discontinuing pacemaker support with various clinical scenarios and the management of potential symptoms.

LVADs

In the setting of mechanical circulatory support, such as LVADs, patients with heart failure are susceptible to death due to cardiovascular causes, device complications and other life-limiting conditions. An increasingly common scenario is the deactivation of LVADs in patients who are not expected to recover or return to a quality of life they consider acceptable.[34] Allen *et al.* suggest that declining quality of life, signs of other organ system failure or an irreversible catastrophic adverse event such as a major stroke or haemorrhage should trigger serious discussions about device deactivation.[26] In a small study of patients with LVADs who elected to discontinue circulatory support, the most common triggers included sepsis, stroke, cancer, renal failure and impending pump failure.[35]

As with other life-prolonging measures such as mechanical ventilation, the discontinuation of an LVAD should only occur after a thorough discussion of burdens, benefits, alternatives and values in a process of informed consent. LVAD deactivation can be performed in the hospital or at home, and requires support from a device-trained individual. As with the withdrawal of any medical therapy, discussions with the patient and family should include consideration of how the device would be stopped, how symptoms would be managed, readiness to proceed and expected outcome.[36] Unlike ICDs, with which deactivation is unlikely to have an immediate effect, LVAD discontinuation can result in rapid decompensation and expected death. The average time to death after device deactivation is approximately 20 minutes, suggesting that careful preparation should be in place prior to device discontinuation. Patients may experience acute pulmonary oedema or thrombosis. LVAD deactivation has been likened to withdrawal of endotracheal intubation and ventilator support and is not an act of physician-assisted suicide or euthanasia, though clinicians' attitudes regarding the ethical issues related to LVAD withdrawal vary.[37] If patients are on multiple forms of advanced life support, a plan is needed to discontinue therapies in a coordinated fashion, provide acute-symptom management and offer acute bereavement support. Potential symptoms following LVAD deactivation may include dyspnoea, anxiety, agitation, pain, noisy breathing and oral secretions. These symptoms can be treated with an opioid and benzodiazepine combination, such as morphine and midazolam titrated to comfort, in a manner similar to mechanical-ventilator withdrawal.[38] Currently, in most areas, it is difficult to coordinate technical expertise for LVAD discontinuation and symptomatic palliation for the dying phase at home or out of the hospital (e.g. nursing home or hospice facility).

PRACTICAL APPROACHES TO CARE FOR THE PATIENT DYING FROM HEART FAILURE

In general, there is a lack of evidence to specifically guide care of the patient dying from heart failure, especially in the last days of life. Clinical trials usually exclude patients estimated to die within 6 months or those with significant renal failure, hypotension or other significant co-morbidities. A consensus statement on palliative and supportive care in advanced heart failure provides a useful summary of clinical recommendations for care of patients with advanced heart failure.[39] Recommendations for this setting can be derived from expert opinion and studies in hospice care which involve patients dying from other illnesses. Practical approaches to the care of the patient dying from heart failure include initial assessment and care, ongoing assessments and care of bereaved family members after death.

Initial assessment

The initial assessment and approach to care should include a review of all medications; a detailed assessment of physical, emotional, social and spiritual needs; and discussion and shared decision-making related to advanced cardiac therapies.

Review all medications and discontinue non-beneficial medications

As the patient approaches the last days of life and enters the active dying phase, medications should be reviewed regularly, as it is usually appropriate to reduce doses or discontinue drugs.[40] Additionally, both cardiac and non-cardiac medications should be reconsidered for whether they are causing, worsening or relieving symptoms due to co-morbidities.[15] The potential impact of medications on delirium or cognitive impairment should be considered, as the risk of impairment is high.

Table 8.3 provides recommendations on conventional medical management in advanced heart failure and the last days of life. Active measures are often continued to aid symptom management, such as diuretics to relieve dyspnoea associated with volume overload. If tolerated and the patient is awake and able to take oral medications, angiotensin-converting enzyme inhibitors and beta-blockers may be continued to prevent worsening heart failure symptoms related to potential increases in blood pressure and sympathetic rebound. Continuing digoxin may provide symptomatic benefit by reducing heart rate and dyspnoea without adversely affecting blood pressure, but, in practice, there is high risk of toxicity related to renal failure.[41] Loop diuretics may be needed until death to help prevent severe pulmonary oedema.[42] Given venous access limitations, furosemide can be administered by intermittent or continuous subcutaneous infusion.[43] Transdermal or buccal nitrates may be useful at this stage, both to relieve angina and, in addition to a loop diuretic, to attempt to prevent pulmonary oedema.

Assess and address physical, emotional, social and spiritual needs

The physical, emotional, social and spiritual needs of the patient dying from advanced heart failure have been introduced earlier in this chapter. Dying patients may experience severe symptoms, including pain, dyspnoea, agitation, nausea and vomiting, and oral secretions. Any symptom should be assessed and managed with a concept of 'total pain' or 'total breathlessness', recognising the need to holistically assess all domains, including physical, psychosocial, spiritual, communication and caregiver needs.[44] Once a symptom related to the active dying phase has been identified, anticipatory or scheduled prescribing of medications should be considered as part of a comprehensive care plan. Table 8.4 provides an overview of good practice points for heart failure patients extrapolated from studies of other terminally ill patients with refractory symptoms.[45] Strategies to manage symptoms should include maximising non-pharmacologic approaches, optimising cardiac management if possible, minimising adverse effects of existing medical therapies, frequent reassessment and a time-limited trial approach. Other non-medical providers and modalities, such as music, art and aromatherapists may play important roles in improving the dying experience.

The approach to the dying patient and family members' psychological, social and spiritual needs requires excellent communication skills and, ideally, should involve an interdisciplinary healthcare team, such as is available through

TABLE 8.3 Recommendations on conventional medical management in advanced heart failure and the last days of life

Medication	Advanced disease	Last days of life*	Considerations
ACE inhibitor	Continue if tolerated	Continue if tolerated	Cough, low BP, high K, renal impairment
Amiodarone	Continue if required for arrhythmia control unless significant adverse effects	Discontinue	Nausea, QT prolongation
Angiotensin receptor blocker	Continue if tolerated	Discontinue	Low BP, high K, renal impairment
Aspirin	Discontinue unless recent infarct	Discontinue	GI irritation and haemorrhage
Beta-blocker	Continue if tolerated	Continue if tolerated	Low HR, Low BP, cold extremities, nightmares, fatigue
Digoxin	Continue if tolerated; requires vigilance to avoid toxicity	Discontinue	Low HR. Risk of toxicity in renal failure (drowsiness, delirium, visual changes, GI symptoms)
Diuretic	Continue with dose titration as required	Continue as needed for symptom relief	Low K, dehydration, gout
Ivabradine	Continue if tolerated	Discontinue	Low HR, visual disturbance, headache
Hydralazine	Continue if tolerated	Discontinue	Low BP, GI disturbance, headache, flushing
Mineralocorticoid receptor antagonist	Continue if tolerated	Discontinue	High K, renal impairment, GI disturbance
Nitrate	Continue if tolerated	Continue as needed for symptom relief	Headache, GI and sleep disturbances
Statin	Discontinue	Discontinue	Myalgia, liver dysfunction

Note: *Oral medications can be continued as indicated and tolerated for symptom relief while the patient remains awake and able to take fluids and medications.
ACE = angiotensin-converting enzyme; BP = blood pressure; GI = gastrointestinal; HR = heart rate; K = potassium.
Source: Adapted from Gadoud *et al.*[45]

hospice care, where the team includes social workers, chaplains, volunteers and others. Effective communication involves responding to emotions;[26,46] discussing serious news, including helping the family understand that the patient is dying; assisting with decision-making regarding advanced cardiac therapies; and approaching existential needs, hopes and fears.[47-9] Family members may

TABLE 8.4 Common symptoms of the active dying phase and suggested approaches to management

Symptom	Medication options	Non-pharmacologic options	Other considerations
Dyspnoea	Opioid Diuretic Nitrate	Hand-held fan; repositioning	Benzodiazepines not recommended as first-line treatment; may be considered if dyspnoea is refractory. Oxygen is not recommended due to uncertain benefit[54]
Pain	Opioid	Target cause if possible; repositioning	Avoid anticholinergic medications (pro-arrhythmogenic) and non-steroidal anti-inflammatory medications (salt and water retention)
Oedema	Diuretic	Watch sodium intake; good skin care	Compression stockings may be burdensome. Refractory ascites may benefit from paracentesis
Anxiety	Benzodiazepine	Emotional support, relaxation techniques	Benzodiazepines may worsen confusion and sedation and pose fall risk
Decreased level of consciousness or delirium	Antipsychotic for agitation or psychosis	Re-orientation, environmental changes (avoid loud noises, display familiar objects and pictures)	Limit vital sign monitoring. If hypoxic, a trial of oxygen therapy for cognitive function
Nausea and vomiting	Anti-emetic	Relaxation techniques, constipation	Avoid strong smells or other triggers
Oral secretions	Anticholinergic	Repositioning; reduce fluid intake	Anticholinergics may be used; however, it is unclear how distressing this symptom is to dying patients. Frequent suctioning is likely to be distressing

Source: Adapted from Gadoud et al.[45] and Adler et al.[55]

struggle with how to inform other individuals of the patient's impending death.

Approaches to social care are closely related to the patient's care location, individual social context and healthcare resources. Family members may need increased practical support and should be connected to available resources, whether in home, hospital or community. The healthcare team should know local programmes and assist with coordination of care. Sensitivity to the patient's cultural and religious background is essential. The healthcare team should explore and support informal or formal religious traditions as part of spiritual care, including identifying whether particular processes should be carried out in the care of the body after death.[50]

Discussion and shared decision-making related to advanced cardiac therapies, especially ICD deactivation

Recognition of the dying phase should lead to communication with the patient and family about appropriate advanced cardiac therapies. For patients in the dying phase, ICD deactivation should be considered to avoid potential shocks. Temporary deactivation can be done by placing a large magnet over the chest wall, but this is only effective while the magnet is present. In a survey of US hospices, only 25% had a magnet available;[28] thus, it is recommended that discussion and plans for deactivation take place early enough to arrange for appropriate technical support. Unlike defibrillation, cardiac resynchronisation therapy has been shown to improve quality of life, so it may be appropriate to continue biventricular pacing even when the decision has been made to inactivate the defibrillator functionality.

Ongoing care of the patient dying of heart failure

The symptom and psychosocial-spiritual burden of patients who are dying may be underappreciated. As such, frequent reassessment is important to providing optimal care. The healthcare team should provide ongoing communication and education to the family regarding what changes may normally occur with dying and how to recognise uncontrolled symptoms or other signs of distress. Family members should be aware of the likelihood of decreasing consciousness and changes in breathing, as well as the potential for audible respiratory secretions and skin changes such as mottling or cyanosis. The healthcare team should provide regular psychological and spiritual support to the patient and family, including identifying issues related to anticipatory grief and individual needs.

A 'good death' cannot be achieved in all patients. Healthcare providers should recognise that suffering cannot always be addressed. Difficult patient or family experiences in the dying phase can be discussed with colleagues to solicit alternative treatment approaches and support. Self-care practices are recommended for providers who frequently care for dying patients.[51]

Care of bereaved family members after death

Regardless of where the patient's death occurs, the healthcare team should be ready to provide support to family members and caregivers immediately after death. Attention should be paid to any special needs or requests for care of the body. Depending on the patient's individual circumstances, it may be appropriate for certain members of the healthcare team to assist with legal or benefit-related issues. If available, information about local resources for bereavement services should be offered to the family. Families should be offered the opportunity to follow up with available resources regarding common emotions or experiences related to bereavement.

SUMMARY

While challenging, recognition of the dying phase is critical to allowing patients with progressive heart failure to experience a supported and symptom-controlled death that aligns with each individual's concept of a good death. As the patient enters the last days of life, there are important opportunities for clear communication to identify the patient's physical, emotional and spiritual needs, as well as the needs of their family or caregivers. The practical approach to the care of the patient dying from heart failure must include a detailed medication review and consideration of deactivation of advanced cardiac therapies (i.e. cardiac devices). While the patient is in the last days of life, the healthcare team should perform frequent and comprehensive symptom assessments and provide attentive symptom management to promote comfort and relief of suffering.

REFERENCES

1 Quill TE. Perspectives on care at the close of life. Initiating end-of-life discussions with seriously ill patients: addressing the 'elephant in the room'. *JAMA*. 2000; **284**(19): 2502–7.

2 Teuteberg J, Teuteberg WG. The course to death in heart failure. In: Beattie J, Goodlin S, editors. *Supportive Care in Heart Failure*. Oxford: Oxford University Press; 2008. pp. 341–63.

3 Steinhauser KE, Christakis NA, Clipp EC *et al*. Factors considered important at the end of life by patients, family, physicians, and other care providers. *JAMA*. 2000; **284**(19): 2476–82.

4 Strachan PH, Ross H, Rocker GM *et al*. Mind the gap: opportunities for improving end-of-life care for patients with advanced heart failure. *Can J Cardiol*. 2009; **25**(11): 635–40.

5 Unroe KT, Greiner MA, Hernandez AF *et al*. Resource use in the last 6 months of life among Medicare beneficiaries with heart failure, 2000–2007. *Arch Intern Med*. 2011; **171**(3): 196–203.

6 www.goldstandardsframework.org.uk/

7 Goldfinger JZ, Adler ED. End-of-life options for patients with advanced heart failure. *Curr Heart Fail Rep*. 2010; **7**(3): 140–7.

8 Morrison RS, Penrod JD, Cassel JB *et al*. Cost savings associated with US hospital palliative care consultation programs. *Arch Intern Med*. 2008; **168**(16): 1783–90.

9 Gadoud A, Kane E, Macleod U et al. Palliative care among heart failure patients in primary care: a comparison to cancer patients using English family practice data. *PLoS One.* 2014; 9(11): e113188.

10 Ellershaw J, Ward C. Care of the dying patient: the last hours or days of life. *BMJ.* 2003; 326(7379): 30–4.

11 Levenson JW, McCarthy EP, Lynn J et al. The last six months of life for patients with congestive heart failure. *J Am Geriatr Soc.* 2000; 48(5 Suppl.): S101–9.

12 Boyd K, Murray SA. Recognising and managing key transitions in end of life care. *BMJ.* 2010; 341: c4863.

13 Bailey FA, Burgio KL, Woodby LL et al. Improving processes of hospital care during the last hours of life. *Arch Intern Med.* 2005; 165(15): 1722–7.

14 Anderson F, Downing GM, Hill J et al. Palliative performance scale (PPS): a new tool. *J Palliat Care.* 1996; 12(1): 5–11.

15 Tevendale E, Baxter J. Heart failure comorbidities at the end of life. *Curr Opin Support Palliat Care.* 2011; 5(4): 322–6.

16 Wilson J, McMillan S. Symptoms experienced by heart failure patients in hospice care. *J Hosp Palliat Nurs.* 2013; 15(1): 13–21.

17 Zambroski CH, Moser DK, Roser LP et al. Patients with heart failure who die in hospice. *Am Heart J.* 2005; 149(3): 558–64.

18 Dougherty CM, Pyper GP, Au DH et al. Drifting in a shrinking future: living with advanced heart failure. *J Cardiovasc Nurs.* 2007; 22(6): 480–7.

19 Hopp FP, Thornton N, Martin L. The lived experience of heart failure at the end of life: a systematic literature review. *Health Soc Work.* 2010; 35(2): 109–17.

20 Molloy GJ, Johnston DW, Witham MD. Family caregiving and congestive heart failure. Review and analysis. *Eur J Heart Fail.* 2005; 7(4): 592–603.

21 Bekelman DB, Nowels CT, Retrum JH et al. Giving voice to patients' and family caregivers' needs in chronic heart failure: implications for palliative care programs. *J Palliat Med.* 2011; 14(12): 1317–24.

22 Small N, Barnes S, Gott M et al. Dying, death and bereavement: a qualitative study of the views of carers of people with heart failure in the UK. *BMC Palliat Care.* 2009; 8: 6.

23 Hunt SA, Abraham WT, Chin MH et al. 2009 Focused update incorporated into the ACC/AHA 2005 Guidelines for the Diagnosis and Management of Heart Failure in Adults: a report of the American College of Cardiology Foundation/American Heart Association Task Force on practice guidelines developed in collaboration with the International Society for Heart and Lung Transplantation. *J Am Coll Cardiol.* 2009; 53(15): e1–90.

24 Kini V, Kirkpatrick JN. Ethical challenges in advanced heart failure. *Curr Opin Support Palliat Care.* 2013; 7(1): 21–8.

25 Wiegand DL, Kalowes PG. Withdrawal of cardiac medications and devices. *AACN Adv Crit Care.* 2007; 18(4): 415–25.

26 Allen LA, Stevenson LW, Grady KL et al. Decision making in advanced heart failure: a scientific statement from the American Heart Association. *Circulation.* 2012; 125(15): 1928–52.

27 Kinch Westerdahl A, Sjöblom J, Mattiasson A-C et al. Implantable cardioverter-defibrillator therapy before death: high risk for painful shocks at end of life. *Circulation.* 2014; 129(4): 422–9.

28 Goldstein N, Carlson M, Livote E *et al.* Brief communication: management of implantable cardioverter-defibrillators in hospice; a nationwide survey. *Ann Intern Med.* 2010; **152**(5): 296–9.

29 Goldstein NE, Lampert R, Bradley E *et al.* Management of implantable cardioverter defibrillators in end-of-life care. *Ann Intern Med.* 2004; **141**(11): 835–8.

30 Hauptman PJ, Swindle J, Hussain Z *et al.* Physician attitudes toward end-stage heart failure: a national survey. *Am J Med.* 2008; **121**(2): 127–35.

31 Strömberg A, Fluur C, Miller J *et al.* ICD recipients' understanding of ethical issues, ICD function, and practical consequences of withdrawing the ICD in the end-of-life. *Pacing Clin Electrophysiol.* 2014; **37**(7): 834–42.

32 Lampert R. Implantable cardioverter-defibrillator shocks in dying patients: disturbing data from beyond the grave. *Circulation.* 2014; **129**(4): 414–16.

33 Mueller PS, Hook CC, Hayes DL. Ethical analysis of withdrawal of pacemaker or implantable cardioverter-defibrillator support at the end of life. *Mayo Clin Proc.* 2003; **78**(8): 959–63.

34 Goldstein NE, May CW, Meier DE. Comprehensive care for mechanical circulatory support: a new frontier for synergy with palliative care. *Circ Heart Fail.* 2011; **4**(4): 519–27.

35 Brush S, Budge D, Alharethi R *et al.* End-of-life decision making and implementation in recipients of a destination left ventricular assist device. *J Heart Lung Transplant.* 2010; **29**(12): 1337–41.

36 Swetz KM, Ottenberg AL, Freeman MR *et al.* Palliative care and end-of-life issues in patients treated with left ventricular assist devices as destination therapy. *Curr Heart Fail Rep.* 2011; **8**(3): 212–18.

37 Swetz KM, Cook KE, Ottenberg AL *et al.* Clinicians' attitudes regarding withdrawal of left ventricular assist devices in patients approaching the end of life. *Eur J Heart Fail.* 2013; **15**(11): 1262–6.

38 von Gunten C, Weissman DE. *Symptom Control for Ventilator Withdrawal in the Dying Patient.* Fast Fact number 34. 2nd ed. 2005. Available at: www.capc.org/fast-facts/34-symptom-control-ventilator-withdrawal-dying-patient/ (accessed 22 May 2015).

39 Goodlin SJ, Hauptman PJ, Arnold R *et al.* Consensus statement: palliative and supportive care in advanced heart failure. *J Card Fail.* 2004; **10**(3): 200–9.

40 Abernethy AP, Kutner J, Blatchford PJ *et al.* Managing comorbidities in oncology: a multisite randomized controlled trial of continuing versus discontinuing statins in the setting of life-limiting illness. *J Clin Oncol.* 2014; **32**(5 Suppl.): abstract LBA9514.

41 Ward C, Dunn FG, Jenkins SM *et al.* Palliative and supportive care for patients with advanced and terminal heart failure. In: Ward C, Witham M, editors. *A Practical Guide to Heart Failure in Older People.* Chichester: Wiley-Blackwell; 2009. pp. 241–70.

42 Faris RF, Flather M, Purcell H *et al.* Diuretics for heart failure. *Cochrane Database Syst Rev.* 2012; **2**: CD003838.

43 Zacharias H, Raw J, Nunn A *et al.* Is there a role for subcutaneous furosemide in the community and hospice management of end-stage heart failure? *Palliat Med.* 2011; **25**(6): 658–63.

44 Abernethy AP, Wheeler JL. Total dyspnoea. *Curr Opin Support Palliat Care.* 2008; **2**(2): 110–13.

45 Gadoud A, Jenkins SM, Hogg KJ. Palliative care for people with heart failure: summary of current evidence and future direction. *Palliat Med.* 2013; **27**(9): 822–8.

46 Tulsky JA. Beyond advance directives: importance of communication skills at the end of life. *JAMA.* 2005; **294**(3): 359–65.

47 Ellershaw J, Johnson M. The last few days of life. In: Beattie J, Goodlin S, editors. *Supportive Care in Heart Failure.* Oxford: Oxford University Press; 2008. pp. 365–76.

48 Back AL, Arnold RM, Quill TE. Hope for the best, and prepare for the worst. *Ann Intern Med.* 2003; **138**(5): 439–43.

49 Quill TE, Arnold RM, Platt F. 'I wish things were different': expressing wishes in response to loss, futility, and unrealistic hopes. *Ann Intern Med.* 2001; **135**(7): 551–5.

50 Neuberger J. *Caring for Dying People of Different Faiths.* 3rd ed. Abingdon, Oxon: Radcliffe Medical Press; 2004.

51 Kearney MK, Weininger RB, Vachon ML *et al.* Self-care of physicians caring for patients at the end of life: 'Being connected . . . a key to my survival'. *JAMA.* 2009; **301**(11): 1155–64.

52 Murray SA, Boyd K, Kendall M *et al.* Dying of lung cancer or cardiac failure: prospective qualitative interview study of patients and their carers in the community. *BMJ.* 2002; **325**(7370): 929.

53 Hansen-Flaschen J. Chronic obstructive pulmonary disease: the last year of life. *Respir Care.* 2004; **49**(1): 90–7; discussion 97–8.

54 Campbell ML, Yarandi H, Dove-Medows E. Oxygen is nonbeneficial for most patients who are near death. *J Pain Symptom Manage.* 2013; **45**(3): 517–23.

55 Adler ED, Goldfinger JZ, Kalman J *et al.* Palliative care in the treatment of advanced heart failure. *Circulation.* 2009; **120**(25): 2597–606.

CHAPTER 9

Palliative care needs of young people with heart failure

HAYLEY PRYSE-HAWKINS AND MIRIAM JOHNSON

INTRODUCTION

Earlier chapters have established that heart failure is a potentially malignant, chronic, debilitating condition affecting a very large number of patients and their families. We have seen that the average age of patients with heart failure in the UK is 77 years, which is similar to the average age of patients with cancer. However, just as with cancer, heart failure can sometimes affect children and young adults, and although the number of such individuals is much smaller, the impact of a life-threatening illness coming early in life can be devastating, and the number living to adulthood but dying as young adults – for example, due to complex congenital heart disease – is increasing.[1]

Little has been written about the specific palliative needs of young people with advanced heart failure, although, in the last few years, the issues experienced by people with end-stage congenital heart disease have been raised.[1-6] Therefore, the approach taken here is largely descriptive rather than based on evidence from the literature. It is important to understand not only what heart failure is but also how it affects people in different stages. For the purpose of this chapter, 'young' will span the years between paediatric and geriatric provision (16–65 years of age). We also deal with more specifically age-related issues, such as sexuality, procreation, body image and transition from paediatric to adult services.

THE NEED FOR EVIDENCE-BASED CARE

To meet the needs of heart failure patients, we will be required to provide evidence of benefit, funding and resources. We need to provide an equitable and inclusive service while being mindful of the individual needs of each patient. Such a service should embrace public and patient involvement and be auditable and adaptable to changing political, cultural and wider service-provisional climates and needs.

As mentioned, heart failure is predominantly a condition of older people and is associated with complex co-morbidities, which may affect quality of life and prognosis equally. Traditionally, research in heart failure used a cohort of people under 70 years old and extrapolated the evidence across the heart failure population. By selecting such subjects, it is generally easier to gain consent, ethical agreement and to avoid confounding from other disease processes. With an older cohort with numerous co-morbidities, it is more difficult to establish the needs and outcomes that are heart failure rather than age specific. For younger patients, there are different problems: for example, the disease processes underlying their heart failure may be very rare, making recruitment difficult for particular aetiologies.

As a result, young people with heart failure will be asked to enter clinical trials and studies at all stages of their disease trajectory, but not always with a potential personal gain. This will require sensitive management and the integration of palliative, cardiac and research services. Young people will need clear guidelines and supportive structures to enable them to partake in such research.

Point to consider

- There is little research specifically into the needs of younger patients with heart failure, despite the high likelihood of young people being involved in research projects.

TIMING OF APPROPRIATE CARE

In contrast with many cancers, in heart failure there is not a clear pathway of care from diagnosis, through treatment, to palliation. Most cardiologists and physicians managing young people with heart failure have little palliative education or experience, and consequently may find it difficult to recognise the needs and transition phases such patients face.

Heart failure patients are more likely to die in hospital and to undergo clinical interventions in the last few weeks and days of their life.[7] This is especially so with younger patients, when hospital staff fail to recognise and accept how close to death patients are. A description of one unit's experience of the circumstances of death, end-of-life discussions and the provision of end-of-life care for 48 patients with congenital heart disease (mean age at death, 37±14 years) reported that most patients had complex congenital heart disease and were considered to be in the end-stage of their disease.[4] Although most were considered by the clinical team to be at end-stage, very few had documented conversations about their preferences and options for end-of-life care prior to their terminal admission, and active and aggressive medical interventions were continued until death for most.[4] Further, a study of the circumstances of death for babies and children with congenital heart disease showed that most died with multi-system failure and receiving highly technical care in the intensive-care unit.[8]

Most health professionals will encounter only a few younger heart failure patients in their working lifetime. A third of patients admitted with decompensated heart failure die within 1 year of their first hospitalisation and up to 50% will be readmitted within the first 6 months after the initial hospitalisation. If palliative care is only to be considered for people within the last year of life, the challenge for health professionals is to identify which patients are more likely to die in the next 12 months. For younger patients, the 'surprise' question (i.e. 'Would you be surprised if this patient died in the next 12 months?') is limited in its usefulness for identifying patients who require palliative care.[9]

Accurately predicting outcomes, disease trajectories and death is difficult for even the most experienced doctor, even without the emotional issues of the patient being as young as or younger than the professional. The emphasis in cardiology care is predominantly curative, and professionals lack the training and support required to recognise the subtle changes that may suggest a patient is dying. There is a fear of recognising and admitting there is no further intervention that can 'save' the patient. There is also a sense of helplessness and ignorance of what happens next among healthcare professionals that make it difficult to recognise and discuss such changes.

We have seen in Chapter 4 that a large number of prognostic tools exists. Cardiac transplant assessments incorporate a variety of these tools and measures to assess suitability for transplantation. These are guides and useful reference points, but, despite intensive monitoring, it is usually difficult to predict which decompensation episode will precede death. However, recognising a change in functional ability, an increasing frequency of decompensation, the need to reduce or stop disease-modifying drugs or an escalation in symptom burden may be a non-invasive prompt to consider supportive care. Staff who are trained and skilled to assess the continually changing needs of their heart failure patients will be better able to recognise when their patients require supportive end-of-life rather than curative care. They will be better able to communicate this to the patient and family and to provide appropriate information, care and resources.

As prognostication appears to be a barrier for clinicians, but less of a concern for patients with regard to the timing of conversations about the end of life, a problem-based approach rather than a prognosis-based approach appears to be more effective. This is consistent with the World Health Organization definition of 'palliative care', which states that palliative care is applicable early on in the disease trajectory alongside active disease-directed treatment.[10]

Emerging work with people with advanced congenital heart disease confirms that such patients wish to be given the opportunity to be involved in decision-making about their future care. A survey of 200 patients identified from the Canadian Adult Congenital Heart Network showed that 85% of service providers were reluctant to initiate discussions about end of life within an estimated 5 years of death, and such prognostication was stated to be difficult – with the effect that such conversations were delayed or avoided.[3] In contrast, 76% of patients, irrespective of disease complexity or stage, said they were ready to discuss end-of-life issues[2] and 78% said they wanted their clinicians to raise the subject.[5] Patients with congenital heart disease have a higher rate of sudden death, leading to calls for end-of-life conversations to be initiated in advance of the onset of heart failure.[6,11] Further, very few (5%) patients had an advance directive in place. Over half (56%) had not heard about the option, but nearly all (87%) stated a preference to have an advance directive available in the event that they were unable to speak for themselves when they were dying.[3] Patients highlighted that the key issues were their trust in their clinicians and their relationship with them – often developed over many years. The authors concluded that end-of-life discussions should not be restricted for those with severely restricted life expectancy.[2]

Points to consider

- Despite heart failure having a poor prognosis, it can be difficult for healthcare professionals to recognise and accept that a young person cannot be cured and is actually dying.
- Most young adults with congenital heart disease would welcome discussions about end-of-life and future care and for their clinicians to raise the subject, even if it is not clear that they are at the end-stage of their disease.

HEALTHCARE-PROFESSIONAL EDUCATION

A palliative care approach, with sensitive discussions and excellent channels of communication, would be helpful for most young heart failure patients and would be best provided by involved heart failure professionals and the primary healthcare team. Many young heart failure patients require access to palliative services at some point, but only a few are likely to need continual access to specialist palliative care professionals. This relies on heart failure and primary care staff education, confidence and collaboration as much as it does on specialist palliative care service provision. The importance of supportive and palliative care for heart failure patients can be seen in the adaptation of the National Institute for Health and Care Excellence guidance.[12,13]

Patients of all ages with heart failure need clear information about heart failure, its symptoms, management and prognosis. They need help and time to understand their disease process, and how this affects them now and in the future. However, whereas some older patients show a preference for letting the doctor take care of their management, most young people wish to understand what may happen next in terms of their symptoms, risks, dependency, treatment and options.[14] This requires a degree of knowledge, experience and openness that is not always easy to find. Heart failure professionals need to have access to education for managing palliative needs and issues, support similar to their palliative colleagues and to adopt an integrated team approach.

Points to consider

- A palliative care approach and skills should be provided by the multidisciplinary and inter-agency healthcare teams involved.
- Involvement by specialist palliative care should only be needed on occasion.
- Education of healthcare professionals in this area is needed.

CARE PATHWAYS

The practical experience of palliative professionals, coupled with an increasingly integrated care pathway, has enabled cancer services to develop models of care that provides an efficient and economic form of service delivery to ensure optimal support and quality of life. Heart failure providers need to review such models and develop similar processes for their patients. A survey of English heart failure nurses found that referrals to palliative care services were facilitated by the presence of formal pathways of care between the two specialties.[15]

Structured pathways of care, using evidence-based protocols and algorithms, may help the healthcare professional to follow a formatted management plan that is individualised to each person. This plan then must be communicated to the patient and their relatives. Following structured pathways of care, or responding to the patient's questions, should highlight the need for further assessment of heart failure status and investigation when symptoms increase despite optimised drug therapy. For the younger patient, this may involve – and, indeed, the patient may often expect – invasive interventions such as cardiac resynchronisation therapy (CRT)[16] or an implantable cardiovertor device,[17] or surgical options such as a left ventricular assist device or cardiac transplantation. Patients are often waiting 'to be sick enough' to have surgery, thinking that if medication is the treatment, surgery is an option saved for the future.

Younger patients tend to be more used to and comfortable with the technical twenty-first century. They are also more likely to use the technical world to help them seek answers for themselves. The Internet is an excellent source of information and support on their health and disease. Unfortunately, not all the information is regulated, and they may access inappropriate information and biased views. Patient and carer expectations and understanding should be reviewed at each clinic visit. Healthcare beliefs and heart failure-specific knowledge should be challenged and information offered and adapted as necessary.

Being considered for invasive intervention suggests the patient has a limited life expectancy and significant morbidity. While the healthcare professional may know this, it needs to be discussed with the patient and relatives, providing a trigger to begin discussions around supportive care and end-of-life decision-making.[18] It needs to be accepted that this is a fluid discussion, and people often change their views as situations change.[19] At present, we have a situation in which patient understanding and consent are routinely required for the process of implementing treatments but not so routinely sought for withdrawing such therapies or for managing end-of-life situations.[20] Patients and relatives should be made aware of the potential benefits and implications of such therapies. Explanation of treatment options should be careful and realistic, and healthcare professionals must address the patient's and relatives' expectations and avoid exaggerated claims of benefit.

Patients and relatives need support during the assessment process and the subsequent wait for treatment. It is especially difficult for patients and relatives waiting for a cardiac transplant.[21,22] The waiting time is indefinable and dependent on the death of another person. Should an organ become available, there is little time to adjust to the idea. Some patients will become too sick to be transplanted or die waiting. Similarly, as the need for CRT increases, the waiting lists will lengthen, too; and since by definition these patients may have a life expectancy of months rather than years, some may die waiting, or not fully benefit from the intervention, because of general associated deterioration. Recent initiatives within the NHS mean that patients with cancer no longer have to wait many weeks or months for investigation and/or treatment. We urgently need similar improvements to service for advanced heart failure, especially in the young. Younger patients and carers are more likely to be aware of, and potentially frustrated by, the economic, political and local variation of service provision. Managing expectation in a media and politically aware group may help to minimise external pressures and stresses.

There are then the patients for who such interventions are not suitable or appropriate.[23] Managing their feelings of rejection, denial or anger takes skill, sensitivity and time. In this process, being honest, consistent and clear, giving people time and permission to explore their fears and feelings in an open and non-threatening or personal manner are essential. Patients and relatives should not feel that they are dismissed with no further options or that palliative and supportive care are adjunct or 'second-best' options; palliative and supportive care are integral to heart failure care, especially at this stage of management. The team supporting such a patient should have access to support and clinical supervision to enhance and sustain such care. Swetz and colleagues found that palliative care consultation along with referral for a left ventricular assist device as destination therapy for people with acquired heart failure resulted in better post-operative care and management of complications.[24] Such an approach will need excellent integrated services and skilled communication between clinicians and with patients with regard to the purpose of the referral.

Another issue that may require sensitive management is that for many young adults with congenital heart disease, there has been a change in the parties involved in decision-making. Whereas their parents were the advocates for care when they were children, it is important that, as young adults, the decision-making becomes patient centred, while acknowledging the distress of their parents and supporting all parties through this transition.[6] Other specialties such as oncology and respiratory medicine face similar challenges with regard to life-limiting diseases of young adults such as cancer or cystic fibrosis, and have described the unique needs of this group of people. Many of these may be applicable to young people with heart disease.[6] Studies with young patients with cancer show that they are more likely to want active participation in conversations about their future care than older adults,[14] leading to calls to ensure a patient-centred rather than parent-centred approach in the clinic.[25]

Increasingly, technology is being used in service delivery, such as 'tele-health' patient monitoring and management programmes. While these may be particularly attractive to younger patients with the added demands of education, work and family commitments, they are often designed with an older, less information technology-experienced patient group in mind. This may make them less user-friendly for this group. Such systems may also concentrate a younger patient group on technological management, with a less focused holistic approach.

Points to consider

- Tailored structured pathways of care can provide a framework for optimising patient management.
- Younger patients are more used to 'technology'.
- Younger patients are more likely to actively seek information.
- Waiting for transplantation or CRT is stressful for patient and carer.
- Patients rejected for intervention must be handled with sensitivity.

RECOGNISING MORTALITY

Death is probably the last taboo in twenty-first century Britain. Consequently, clear and open communication regarding prognosis and end-of-life issues is not provided for many people with heart failure, particularly the younger patient.

There is one factor common to all humans, and that is we shall all die. How and when is unknown to most of us, and is generally not something we often contemplate.

Many young people have not had exposure to death and grief. Lacking exposure to the processes and language associated with dying, they have not developed their own coping mechanisms. Older generations frequently have some experience and understanding of death – from war experiences through to family and friends. Many older people will talk about their peers being ill and dying. There is frequently an acceptance that they have lived and are nearing death, even though this may be an abstract acceptance. A lack of death or grieving experience and vocabulary may make it difficult for the younger patient to introduce the subject, and, as such, they may also miss the healthcare professional's probing questions.

Older people have often reached a reflective phase of their life, while very young people are in the planning phases of life. Older people have experiences and memories to look back on; they have an identity and achievements to reflect on. Young people have few achievements or memories, and often have not established their identity yet. Lost time, experiences and achievements should be recognised, and permission to grieve for these may be required. Less experience means they may also have less understanding of the mechanics of the healthcare system.

Young people frequently do not expect to die prematurely, even though they may know and understand their diagnosis.[26] This makes discussing the potential of sudden death particularly difficult; indeed, young people often have difficulty recognising and accepting they will die at any stage. They cannot imagine not being part of life or how to plan for their future and that of their family and friends. There is frequently a great deal of anger associated with the diagnosis and prognosis. It is difficult for family and friends to recognise and accept that this is a terminal condition and there are no cures. Young people need to recognise and accept their dying state to plan for, and gain some sense of control over, their death. They may need practical help to write a will, get their affairs in order and make funeral arrangements.

Unrealistic expectations and denial can mean that family and friends find it difficult to cope with the present situation and ignore the future changes required. This deprives the young heart failure patient of valuable and necessary support and assistance, both physical and psychosocial. Confusion and lack of clarity about the disease trajectory and prognosis is common, unsettling and difficult to cope with, and this exacerbates the feelings of uselessness, denial and unrealistic expectation. Younger heart failure patients may have different understanding and expectations regarding their trajectories, so clarification should be sought, documented and reviewed regularly.

Young people lack not only experience of illness and death but also the culture and language of death. This makes it particularly difficult for patients to recognise and express their needs, fears and anxieties, which in turn can make it difficult for family and friends to communicate effectively with them. This can lead to isolation and feelings of rejection, as peers avoid contact because they 'do not know what to say' or are afraid of the personal and unsettling feelings the patients' illness stimulates. Fear of illness and death may be acute and disabling in peers and may increase sensations of unfairness and helplessness.[27]

Such confusion and fears are played out in a culture of 'immediate sharing' in the remote environment of social media. This may be enabling and liberating but can also enhance vulnerability. Such young people are often exploring who they are, may not have a secure network of support and may be confused about their spirituality and beliefs, all of which may increase their sense of isolation and vulnerability. Chaplaincy services are a useful resource but may not be immediately identified as a resource to, or for, the young.

Points to consider

- Younger patients do not expect a premature death, even if they know and understand their diagnosis.
- Younger patients may have little experience or language of dying.

UNDERSTANDING HEART FAILURE

There is widespread knowledge and acceptance of cancer, its treatment options and prospect of death. Many people will know of someone who has or had cancer. This is often not the case with heart failure. Its treatment and effects are generally not well understood by the general public. This can make it difficult for friends, neighbours and society to understand the needs of people with heart failure, and this, in turn, can lead to a feeling of frustration and isolation. The need to explain their illness and symptoms often means that people avoid discussing their heart failure with people other than their immediate family and healthcare professionals.

This may mean that young people with heart failure are more dependent on healthcare professionals for information, support and the ability to discuss their fears and concerns.[28,29] Many will wait for the professionals to raise issues around death, coping and end of life. To tackle this difficult agenda, professionals require support and training, and the confidence to become more proactive in encouraging young patients to discuss difficult issues. If patients are to accept their diagnosis and prognosis and achieve a reasonable quality of life, they and their carers will also need information and support.[26,28] There needs to be a shift in emphasis from the medical model towards a practical, psychosocial strategy, implementing more holistic care.

PHYSICAL NEEDS

Young people will often not highlight needs, because they do not wish to accept that they exist or that they are irreversible. Physical needs are often linked to medication, with symptoms being confused with side effects of drugs – or belief that the medication is not working and asking for further interventions. If the physical symptoms and altered functional needs are assessed and addressed early, many can be minimised and stabilised for longer periods, thus improving quality of life.

To ensure the appropriate information and support are delivered at the pace and level required, assessments and evaluation of needs are required at frequent intervals. The UK Single Assessment Process policy should ensure an initial comprehensive assessment of physical and psychosocial needs. However, this does not obviate the need for regular follow-up, and clear and timely communication is mandatory between all associated health- and social care professionals and agencies.

Younger people have particular difficulty in accepting many physical symptoms associated with reduced functional capacity, and this has an impact on quality of life. A slower pace and being breathless when running for a bus, climbing stairs or walking up a slope may be viewed as part of the ageing process and therefore tolerated as inevitable in older patients. This is not so with younger people, who may be acutely embarrassed by such signs and therefore avoid activities that further restrict their functional capacity, and this can lead to social isolation and depression. Such functional changes highlight they are different from their peers, and being different is often not acceptable to the young.

EXERCISE AND ACTIVITY

Exercise is an essential component of physical and mental health. An inability to exercise regularly therefore impairs such health. Young people need access to advice on how to exercise to improve their physical and mental health and to delay the development of heart failure and death. Access to cardiac rehabilitation programmes is rare for young people with heart failure. There are very few rehabilitation programmes specifically for heart failure, and some cardiac rehabilitation programmes will not accept heart failure referrals. People who have heart failure secondary to ischaemic heart disease may get access to rehabilitation programmes, but these are generally in older age groups.

Exercise training should be commenced on diagnosis, and young people tend to be working or studying at this point. They may not have sufficient time and energy to manage day-to-day living, and so may reduce exercise because they link the tiredness and breathlessness associated with exercise to their disease. The benefits of exercise, together with practical guidelines on how to do it, need to be available and reiterated frequently. The National Institute for Health and Care Excellence guidelines on heart failure state that patients need access to informed support on exercise, but not all clinicians have the knowledge, experience or confidence to educate their patients.[13]

Exercise training and guidance may improve quality of life and delay functional deterioration but must not be viewed in isolation. Access to gyms and exercise classes may be more the norm to younger generations, but young people may need to discuss practical implications, such as time, cost, pacing themselves and body image, first. An acceptance of their present level of fitness and function is required, with an understanding of what to expect. Setting small realistic goals in exercise training will encourage engagement and improve chances of success.

Healthcare professionals should be mindful of the associated sensitivities that exercise raises in the younger person. Exercise is often associated with looks, physique, body image, fitness and 'pumping iron' and may introduce an element of competition and inequality that heightens feelings of inadequacy and low self-esteem.

> **Points to consider**
>
> - Exercise training improves quality of life and delays functional deterioration.
> - Younger patients may feel self-conscious about body image, so be reluctant to join a gymnasium.

PHYSICAL SUPPORT

Young patients often find it difficult to access timely physical support. Older people will often have their physical daily needs assessed – because of their age if not their diagnosis. Younger patients are often not identified and therefore do not benefit from care bundles and regular reviews. There is a general assumption that young people can self-care, with the result that their daily needs are not noted in hospital or the outpatient setting. It is assumed that, because you are young, you can cope without help. As we get older, we often slowly learn to adapt physically and emotionally to altering physical function, and these adaptations and coping mechanisms are often shared within our peer group. This is not the case with younger patients. Information and advertisements regarding equipment generally feature older people, making it appear less attainable and attractive to younger people.

Young people are often confused, frustrated and angry at their reduced functional ability. They may see their reduced function as a failure of the treatment not progression of the condition. Explaining the disease trajectory and addressing expectations may enable the individual to accept, adapt and cope better, enhancing the patient's experience, satisfaction and quality of life.

Physical activities may be used to manage and relieve stress. Being unable to partake of these activities adds stress and disables previous coping mechanisms. Addressing stress management is an important aspect of care for the younger patient.

Honest and open discussion of individual physical needs encourages long-term engagement. If periodic reviews are built into heart failure management, it then becomes easier to identify changes and manage these effectively. However, recognising the needs is only part of the problem; heart failure professionals should be aware of the services available within their community and how to access them.

MULTI-AGENCY WORKING

Effective care for heart failure patients of any age requires an integrated multi-agency approach: engaging, educating and supporting colleagues in a variety of settings. It requires advanced communication, an openness and willingness to share experiences and learn from and with each other and an ability to raise the profile of heart failure and its effects on patients and their carers. Heart failure patients need access to personal and domestic care and financial and social support, irrespective of age. It is vital to avoid confusion and duplication by including all parties relevant and important to the patient and to have a designated key worker.

The culture of increasingly long working days, with immediate, 24/7 availability in the workplace makes it difficult for the working patient with heart failure to compete and maintain a healthy work–life balance. A changing political and social agenda, debated and popularised in parts of the media, encourages work as the accepted norm and portrays the claiming of benefits as unacceptable. Therefore, it is important that such changing needs in younger patients be assessed and addressed by the healthcare professional.

Professional awareness and help to complete care and benefit forms minimise a daunting, confusing and often humiliating task.[30] Such forms generally do not lend themselves to recognising and capturing the needs of young people and their fluctuating personal, physical, mental and social needs.

Eligibility for NHS-funded continuing care is reliant on individual healthcare needs assessment, not diagnosis or exact life expectancy. Patients should not be exempt because a clear life expectancy cannot be guesstimated. Not all heart failure professionals are aware of the DS1500 form (which accelerates benefit claims for ill patients) or may not feel confident to complete the form in case the patient does not die within 6 months. Access to informed staff who are able to keep abreast of changing benefit and social-care rules is the essential requirement to ensuring patients are able to choose where they wish to live and die.

Points to consider

- Work, education and work–life balance may be additional stresses for young people, which need to be sensitively assessed and discussed.
- Young people need access to the personal and domestic care and financial help but this is often overlooked.
- Multi-agency support is required to find social and financial solutions.

FAMILY AND CARERS

The needs of older people are obvious and accepted by other health, social-services and voluntary agencies, but not so those of the younger heart failure patient, which therefore frequently go unmet. The burden of care frequently falls upon parents, children, partners and others, who often do not identify themselves as 'carers'. A spouse or child will frequently adjust to changing circumstances within the home, adopting a variety of tasks and roles previously held by the patient. This can have a dramatic impact on relationships and family dynamics.

The needs of carers are acknowledged in the Carers (Equal Opportunities) Act 2004, but the practicalities involved in addressing their needs are frequently ignored or under-resourced. The Census 2001[31] suggested that 1 in 10 of the population in England and Wales are carers. Carers frequently state that the ability to have a break is the most significant support they require. There is a gap in the commissioning and provision of respite facilities for this younger group, for who nursing-home respite care may not be available or appropriate. Heart failure professionals need access to information regarding such available resources, and there should be recognition of the impact of heart failure on patients and their carers. Greater research on the daily reality of living with young people with heart failure will enhance understanding and recognition.

Young carers can experience a protracted grieving process while their loved one dies slowly of heart failure. In addition, as implied earlier, when a spouse becomes a carer, this subtly changes the balance of the relationship. The increasing physical, mental and emotional strain experienced by the carer is often not noted or acknowledged by the patient, carer, family and healthcare professionals. This can result in carer and patient unmet needs, frustrations, isolation and impaired or maladaptive coping mechanisms. In both the short- and long-term, this will affect how they cope, feel and how patients perceive and accept their diagnosis and prognosis.

Time is important when the future is unsure; emotional concerns and needs are rarely given priority over physical tasks. Accessing physical support in the form of personal care, housework or shopping can relieve the carer to engage in more positive activities like organising a social gathering or simply give them the time to enjoy a movie together. For many, the extended period of uncertainty in heart failure means lives are put on hold, and the emotional and physical stresses and tension are experienced for a longer period than with most cancers.

It can be particularly hard for parents to have an increasingly dependent child who is a young adult. It comes at a stage when their peers' children are leaving home, settling down and starting families of their own, free from child-care responsibilities. On a physical level, it can be hard to go back to disturbed nights, basic hygiene care and lifting a heavy adult when no longer young themselves. On a psychological level, it is hard to deal with the loss of the child's future, potential grandchildren and the fulfilment of achievement. There are inevitable worries about what may happen to their child should they become ill, die or less able to cope physically, mentally or emotionally as they age. There are financial implications for the ageing carer of a child, as their income decreases and they cannot realise accrued financial assets, which many of their peers may enjoy. For the patient, it can be hard to be cared for again by the parent, often after a period of independence, and they may feel as if they are a young child again or a burden.

> **Points to consider**
>
> - Illness creates tensions and changes in roles within families.
> - Carers become exhausted and respite care is difficult to find for the younger patient.
> - When a young adult is being cared for by parents, this can cause particular strain on the parent–child relationship.

SEXUAL NEEDS

We all need to be and feel loved. A lack of personal physical contact can be distressing to all family members but to partners especially. We are sexual beings, and our sexual needs are no less important because we are ill and dying. It may be difficult for parents caring for their child to recognise or discuss such needs.

There are physical and emotional reasons why people with heart failure experience sexual problems. The most obvious issue is a lack of energy and functional ability. People who are used to exercising regularly and able to tolerate a degree of breathlessness through training will manage the physical concerns better. Discussing the issue and practical solutions – like resting and avoiding heavy meals prior to sexual intercourse and trying different positions – can help. Impaired cardiac output affects the blood supply to the skin and sexual organs, which can result in impaired sensation and pleasure and the ability to have or maintain an erection. Drugs can further affect this through their side effects, effect on lowering blood pressure or effect on the mucous membranes (diuretics). Moreover, depression, low self-esteem and altered body image may affect libido. An assessment of sexual function and need is a delicate task and is often not performed regularly but can be linked to discussion of exercise, drug therapy and psychosocial well-being.

Sexual and sensual pleasure is not confined to penetration. Recognising and discussing needs can help find alternative ways to provide sexual pleasure. Fears, frustrations, misunderstandings and expectations can unnecessarily restrict sexual activity. Patients and partners need to understand and accept the diagnosis and reality of life with heart failure. Fears about physical ability and risk should be sensitively explored and challenged. Practical suggestions regarding minimising exertion are important factors to easing this embarrassing subject. Positions that require supporting the body through the arms may not be realistic in many patients who have weak and cachexic arm muscles. This weakness can also inhibit masturbation. Very close intimate contact can be uncomfortable and claustrophobic to the breathless patient. Partners' fears of physical symptoms and 'what if' scenarios often limit and restrict sexual experiences and pleasure.

Apart from the natural fear of embarrassment, professionals may avoid raising the subject of sexual needs because of their lack of knowledge and resources for managing issues. Access to erectile-dysfunction clinics and materials as well as relationship and sexual counselling should be available to heart failure teams to empower them to assess and meet such needs.

Points to consider

- Sexual contact is often important.
- Assessment can be broached in the context of psychosocial well-being.

BODY IMAGE

Heart failure can seriously affect one's body image, which, in turn, can affect one's self-confidence, sexuality, mood and willingness to self-care. Women with heart failure are frequently heard to lament 'the loss of the only thin part of them' as they look at their swollen ankles. Heart failure and its management can cause swollen ankles, a distended abdomen, muscle loss, thinning and dry skin, peeling lips, altered colour (including jaundice, blue lips, white/blue peripheries, red and weeping cellulitic legs, red/brown chronically engorged legs); alopecia, gynaecomastia, dry, irritating cough; and a runny nose – to mention just a few of the frustrating and inconvenient physical characteristics. Physical appearance is important to all humans, being part of our identity. Such physical characteristics and limitations (e.g. peripheral coolness, postural dizziness and urinary frequency) affect our choice of clothes, shoes, activities and social interactions. This is a major handicap for young single people who wish to interact with their peers and seek opportunities to meet new friends and potential partners.

THE NEED TO PROCREATE

Sexual intercourse is not simply a physical and emotional need; there is the need in all of us to procreate. The wish to have a child is universally acknowledged but may be impossible for a young person with heart failure. Such a missed opportunity can have a significant impact on the emotional well-being of the patient and their partner. It leads to feelings of inadequacy, failure, frustration and depression. The need to have a child is linked to our sense of the continuity of life, and the realisation that when we die we will leave nothing of ourselves behind is difficult to cope with. This can have serious effects on relationships and is especially difficult to manage in some ethnic cultures in which procreation is an essential part of marriage and identity.

Informed heart failure staff should discuss the implications and risks associated with having a child with access to associated services. Men with heart failure who wish to have a child need to explore the physical possibilities of impregnating their partner. If maintaining an erection is difficult, guidance regarding erectile aides and suitable positions that minimise effort and function for the man need to be discussed. It is important to remember that drugs such as sildenafil (Viagra®) lower the blood pressure and may require several doses over time to reach optimal effect. If such physical effort or erectile function is not possible, alternative services such as IVF may be considered.

The physical effects associated with pregnancy and delivery make pregnancy for some women with heart failure inadvisable. The potential effects on the mother and foetus (from drugs especially) should be sensitively and explicitly explored with both partners. In the few cases when pregnancy does occur, specialist antenatal and postnatal care should be accessed immediately. The risks of planned or spontaneous termination and the risks of birth defects should be discussed. Collaborating with local 'high-risk' maternity services will ensure access to appropriate support, investigations and management. Pharmacists and adult congenital heart disease services are invaluable resources and sources of information.

Therefore, it is essential that the topic be raised with all heart failure patients of childbearing age and that methods of contraception be discussed. There are limited contraceptive choices available to women with heart failure. The thromboembolic risks associated with the contraceptive pill make this an unattractive and inadvisable method. The sheath is often not a practical option due to the other physical limitations associated with sexual intercourse for people with heart failure, and its relatively poor reliability makes it an undesirable choice when pregnancy is absolute contraindicated. Heart failure professionals may need to work with contraceptive services to offer the support and advice necessary to couples.

Such coordinated working is also required to address the genetic issues that patients with familial or idiopathic cardiomyopathy face. Information regarding genetic counselling, family screening and linking to paediatric cardiac services should be available and discussed with parents and couples planning a family. The practical concerns of raising a family should be discussed, such as financial and child-care constraints. Parents need to be aware of what services and information they can access for practical parenting issues and how to plan for the future with their children.

The individual and specific needs of women whose heart failure aetiology is peri- or postpartum should be explored and recognised. Linking in with the general practitioner and health visitor will provide additional practical and emotional support. Coping with a chronic or terminal condition while adjusting to having a child is difficult for parents.

Points to consider

- Men may need guidance regarding erectile dysfunction.
- Women need specialist pre-/ante-/postnatal care if they wish to become pregnant.
- Counselling is required about the risk of birth defects and the cardiovascular risk of pregnancy.
- Collaborative working with specialist congenital heart disease and specialised

cardiomyopathy services may be beneficial for the local heart failure community, and associated professionals.

NEEDS OF CHILDREN

Children especially find it difficult to cope with a parent being chronically ill and dying. The needs of children may be ignored because of fears of the professional and patient as to how to address them sensitively. Heart failure professionals who honestly engage in discussions about end of life and supportive care are likely to identify such needs. It is important to access the appropriate training and resources to cope with such complex emotional needs. Being aware of the wider healthcare team enables contact with school nurses, health visitors, professional counselling and bereavement services, social workers and paediatric services.

Not being there for their children in the future is a major concern of dying parents. This fear should be addressed and practical suggestions explored to help them cope and feel part of their child's future, such as writing letters, making tapes or videos, leaving treasured personal belongings and making plans for their education or holidays. Some parents compile photo albums, music recordings and make or buy gifts to be given to their children in the future.

Heart failure patients may have younger siblings who need to be considered within the family dynamics. Their experiences, fears and needs should be sensitively explored and bereavement risk assessed.

Point to consider

- Younger patients may have young children who will therefore lose a parent at a young age.

TRANSITION

Survivorship is currently a key theme in cancer care. With improvements in research and therapies, many children are surviving childhood cancers. Due to their past treatments, some of these survivors are now developing heart failure. Adolescents with cancer are also developing therapy-related heart failure. The number of young people surviving complex congenital heart conditions through childhood but going on to develop heart failure later is a growing group with individual physical and psychological needs. Adult services need to be aware of the developmental and psychological needs of this specific group of 17- to 24-year-olds.

Many children make the transition from paediatric to adult services with a lack of coordination between relevant agencies and little or no involvement from the young person or their family. There is inadequate planning and communication, which leads to despondency, frustration and potentially lost opportunities. Uniform access to integrated service provision would minimise confusion and sudden loss of support and services.

The family is a key consideration in managing children with a terminal illness. Family and personal carers do not necessarily have the same recognition or available support in young-adult services. Parents often have difficulty adapting to the changing needs and responsibilities of a well adolescent, and this can be additionally complex when they are sick and dying. The needs of children are paramount in paediatric palliative care services, and experiences and knowledge may be shared to enhance and develop heart failure palliative care services for young people

The transition from paediatric to adult services is a growing area that is in need of exploration to influence future service development. The needs of both the patient and their family require careful assessment and planning. The philosophy and expectations of paediatric and adult services vary considerably, and they are frequently separated geographically. A coordinated approach, from commissioning to service development, implementation, training and audit, is essential.

END-OF-LIFE CHOICES

The UK government's independent report on choice in end of life care[32] encompasses equity and responsive care provision to individual needs and requires resources and an empowered patient to work. The language associated with palliative and supportive care is unfamiliar to many and can increase confusion and distress unless broached with sensitivity. The terms 'palliative care' and 'hospice' are emotive and can adversely influence patients' acceptance of services, with many believing that hospice care involves stopping all medication and giving-in to death. It is important to generate discussion around their understandings, misunderstandings, beliefs and expectations.

Discussions with patients and families about palliative and hospice care can be difficult for even the most experienced professional. Planning the transition to palliative or supportive care begins with exploring and accepting the patient's and family's understanding of heart failure, prognosis, expectations, fears and wishes. Using questions that facilitate and encourage discussion of such emotional needs in a safe environment, avoiding emotive terminology, encourages acceptance of some of the issues and changes the focus from treating the disease to living and coping with the disease.

An early acceptance of the potentially terminal nature of the condition, with an understanding of the practical implications, prepares people for the future. Practical and ethical decisions made and understood make the end-of-life period less traumatic. Access to acceptable, appropriate and realistic service provision facilitates choice in place of care and death for more people. It ensures clarity between all service providers and family members, preventing unrealistic expectations and demands, unwanted admissions and clinical interventions. Clear instructions of what to do and who to contact in particular situations enhance carers' sense of control and comfort. It is important that carers and families recognise their own emotional and physical needs in the dying phase. Failure to do so can make bereavement and recovery after the patient's death difficult.

The financial stresses for people living with, and dying from, a chronic condition are often considerable and an added burden. Evidence-based drug therapy means young heart failure patients will be taking, and paying for, a minimum of three medications. With medication to minimise the associated symptoms of the condition, this increases significantly, which is an important financial consideration that cancer patients do not experience, as they receive free prescriptions. While a prepaid prescription certificate will reduce such a cost annually, it is a large sum to pay in one go.

Preparing and planning for the future may be difficult and emotional for patients, carers and healthcare professionals, but it may also minimise stress and uncertainty. Discussions around prognosis and increasing symptom burden may prompt a patient to take early retirement and improve their quality of life. Young patients may wish to reduce monthly costs by stopping payments into life-insurance policies and pensions and cash them in, if appropriate. Financial planning is influenced by life expectancy, and young people should be enabled to make appropriate decisions.

'What if' questions can be a focus for exploring fears and potential scenarios, which may help to inform choices regarding preferred place of care and death, and planning advance directives.[31]

Education and training in palliation and clinical supervision are not routinely recognised as fundamental for the heart failure team, thus are not comprehensively available or funded. Enabling a team to recognise and discuss these important aspects of care, in abstract, academically and as a focus of service provision, may improve care for the individual patient, while reducing fears and stresses for healthcare professionals when managing the dying patient.

Point to consider

- Sensitive communication is key to allowing patient choice with regard to end-of-life care.

PUBLIC AND USER INVOLVEMENT

Public and user involvement is currently a political driving force in healthcare provision strategy. It provides an excellent opportunity for patients and their carers to share their experiences, highlight needs and shape the future for heart failure care.

Such involvement requires the trust and recognition of the value of the patient's involvement and is dependent on the patient having a sense of control of their heart failure management. Informed patients empowered and supported to self-care on diagnosis, with access to appropriately trained and skilled integrated multidisciplinary teams, should not need access to specialist palliative services routinely. This should remove the uncertainty and confusion surrounding referrals, ensuring people have access to supportive and practical help when they most need it and so they are able to readily access their right of choice to their place of living and dying.

SUMMARY

Specific evidence from randomised clinical trials may not be available for managing young people with palliative heart failure needs, but there are patients in this group needing care now. The available evidence shows a group of people who die receiving aggressive therapy and who have little involvement in decisions regarding their end-of-life care, despite a willingness to do so and an expectation that their trusted healthcare professionals will initiate the discussion. The challenge is to identify, extrapolate and reflect on available evidence, models and healthcare systems or structures and marry these to the needs of young people with end stage heart failure. Integrated care teams that actively seek patient and family involvement, honest and open communication, and manage and reflect on expectation will support and educate not only the patient and family but also team members. The authors hope that this chapter will encourage the range of professionals involved in caring for younger patients with heart failure to meet this challenge.

REFERENCES

1 Greutmann M, Tobler D, Kovacs AH et al. Increasing mortality burden among adults with complex congenital heart disease. *Congenit Heart Dis.* 2015; **10**(2): 117–27.

2 Greutmann M, Tobler D, Colman JM et al. Facilitators of and barriers to advance care planning in adult congenital heart disease. *Congenit Heart Dis.* 2013; **8**(4): 281–8.

3 Tobler D, Greutmann M, Colman JM et al. Knowledge of and preference for advance care planning by adults with congenital heart disease. *Am J Cardiol.* 2012; **109**(12): 1797–800.

4 Tobler D, Greutmann M, Colman JM et al. End-of-life care in hospitalized adults with complex congenital heart disease: care delayed, care denied. *Palliat Med.* 2012; **26**(1): 72–9.

5 Tobler D, Greutmann M, Colman JM et al. End-of-life in adults with congenital heart disease: a call for early communication. *Int J Cardiol.* 2012; **155**(3): 383–7.

6 Bowater SE, Speakman JK, Thorne SA. End-of-life care in adults with congenital heart disease: now is the time to act. *Curr Opin Support Palliat Care.* 2013; **7**(1): 8–13.

7 Lynn J, Teno JM, Phillips RS et al. Perceptions by family members of the dying experience of older and seriously ill patients. SUPPORT Investigators. Study to Understand Prognoses and Preferences for Outcomes and Risks of Treatments. *Ann Intern Med.* 1997; **126**(2): 97–106.

8 Morell E, Wolfe J, Scheurer M *et al*. Patterns of care at end of life in children with advanced heart disease. *Arch Pediatr Adolesc Med*. 2012; **166**(8): 745–8.

9 Haga K, Murray S, Reid J *et al*. Identifying community based chronic heart failure patients in the last year of life: a comparison of the Gold Standards Framework Prognostic Indicator Guide and the Seattle Heart Failure Model. *Heart*. 2012; **98**(7): 579–83.

10 World Health Organization (WHO). *WHO Definition of Palliative Care*. Geneva: WHO; nd. Available at: www.who.int/cancer/palliative/definition/en/ (accessed 23 May 2015).

11 Tobler D, de SN, Greutmann M. Supportive and palliative care for adults dying from congenital heart defect. *Curr Opin Support Palliat Care*. 2011; **5**(3): 291–6.

12 NHS. *National Service Framework for Coronary Heart Disease: modern standards and service models*. London: Department of Health; 2000. Available at: www.gov.uk/government/uploads/system/uploads/attachment_data/file/198931/National_Service_Framework_for_Coronary_Heart_Disease.pdf (accessed 23 May 2015).

13 National Institute for Health and Clinical Excellence. *Chronic Heart Failure: management of chronic heart failure in adults in primary and secondary care*. NICE guideline CG108. London: National Institute for Health and Clinical Excellence; 2010. www.nice.org.uk/guidance/CG108

14 Brown VA, Parker PA, Furber L *et al*. Patient preferences for the delivery of bad news – the experience of a UK cancer centre. *Eur J Cancer Care (Engl)*. 2011; **20**(1): 56–61.

15 Johnson MJ, MacCallum A, Butler J *et al*. Heart failure specialist nurses' use of palliative care services: a comparison of surveys across England in 2005 and 2010. *Eur J Cardiovasc Nurs*. 2011; **11**(2): 190–6.

16 Linde C, Leclercq C, Rex S *et al*. Long-term benefits of biventricular pacing in congestive heart failure: results from the MUltisite STimulation in cardiomyopathy (MUSTIC) study. *J Am Coll Cardiol*. 2002; **40**(1): 111–18.

17 Young JB, Abraham WT, Smith AL *et al*. Combined cardiac resynchronization and implantable cardioversion defibrillation in advanced chronic heart failure: the MIRACLE ICD Trial. *JAMA*. 2003; **289**(20): 2685–94.

18 Berger JT. The ethics of deactivating implanted cardioverter defibrillators. *Ann Intern Med*. 2005; **142**(8): 631–4.

19 Krumholz HM, Phillips RS, Hamel MB *et al*. Resuscitation preferences among patients with severe congestive heart failure: results from the SUPPORT project. Study to Understand Prognoses and Preferences for Outcomes and Risks of Treatments. *Circulation*. 1998; **98**(7): 648–55.

20 Goldstein NE, Lampert R, Bradley E *et al*. Management of implantable cardioverter defibrillators in end-of-life care. *Ann Intern Med*. 2004; **141**(11): 835–8.

21 Evangelista LS, Dracup K, Moser DK *et al*. Two-year follow-up of quality of life in patients referred for heart transplant. *Heart Lung*. 2005; **34**(3): 187–93.

22 Castle H, Jones I. A long wait: how nurses can help patients through the transplantation pathway. *Prof Nurse*. 2004; **19**(12): 37–9.

23 Jaarsma T, Beattie JM, Ryder M *et al*. Palliative care in heart failure: a position statement from the palliative care workshop of the Heart Failure Association of the European Society of Cardiology. *Eur J Heart Fail*. 2009; **11**(5): 433–43.

24 Swetz KM, Freeman MR, AbouEzzeddine OF *et al*. Palliative medicine consultation

for preparedness planning in patients receiving left ventricular assist devices as destination therapy. *Mayo Clin Proc.* 2011; **86**(6): 493–500.

25 Freyer DR. Transition of care for young adult survivors of childhood and adolescent cancer: rationale and approaches. *J Clin Oncol.* 2010; **28**(32): 4810–18.

26 Murray SA, Boyd K, Kendall M *et al.* Dying of lung cancer or cardiac failure: prospective qualitative interview study of patients and their carers in the community. *BMJ.* 2002; **325**(7370): 929.

27 Hynson JL, Gillis J, Collins JJ *et al.* The dying child: how is care different? *Med J Aust.* 2003; **179**(6 Suppl.): S20–2.

28 Mårtensson J, Karlsson JE, Fridlund B. Male patients with congestive heart failure and their conception of the life situation. *J Adv Nurs.* 1997; **25**(3): 579–86.

29 Mårtensson J, Karlsson JE, Fridlund B. Female patients with congestive heart failure: how they conceive their life situation. *J Adv Nurs.* 1998; **28**(6): 1216–24.

30 Ward C. Improving access to financial support for heart failure patients: understanding the claims process and the doctor's role. *Br J Cardiol.* 2007; **14**(5): 275–9.

31 Candy B, Jones L, Drake R *et al.* Interventions for supporting informal caregivers of patients in the terminal phase of a disease. *Cochrane Database Syst Rev.* 2011; (6): CD007617.

CHAPTER 10

Palliative care services for patients with heart failure

MIRIAM JOHNSON, NATHAN GOLDSTEIN, LAURA GELFMAN, PIOTR SOBANSKI, PATRICIA DAVIDSON, JANE PHILLIPS AND PHILIP NEWTON

INTRODUCTION

As the broader needs of patients with heart failure become more widely recognised (*see* Chapter 1, 'The need for palliative care in heart failure'), so further challenges arise – how best to provide the supportive and palliative care that is so clearly needed, and what the specific role of specialist palliative care (SPC) services should be. This chapter discusses some of the barriers to SPC involvement, and offers views from the UK, Continental Europe, the USA and Australia describing the extent to which people with heart failure are able to access such care.

GENERIC SUPPORTIVE AND PALLIATIVE CARE SERVICES

The importance of generic palliative care skills has been emphasised throughout this book. 'Generic palliative care' is that which should be provided by all healthcare workers, irrespective of specialty and setting, acknowledging that specialist services never can provide all the palliative care for all who need it.[1] The principles of symptom control based on a holistic assessment that includes physical, psychological and spiritual domains should be familiar to all health professionals who should be able to deal with all but complex issues. Increasingly, nursing staff in particular are becoming aware of patient needs in these areas, and heart failure nurse specialists (HFNSs), district nurses, practice nurses (who have often gained great skill in running chronic disease-management clinics) and community matrons can play an important role in coordinating care. Most general practitioners will be involved with patients who have advanced heart failure and have experience of palliative care, but their skills relating to advanced heart failure may be variable.

In primary care, the Macmillan Gold Standards Framework[2] (GSF) provides a standardised organisational framework of multi-professional care. Although it was first developed for palliative care needs for cancer patients, it is largely also applicable to non-cancer patients. It continues to be used by many general practices in the UK and fosters a consistent palliative approach for patients who are likely to be in their last 6–12 months of life. Emphasis is placed on coordination of care, anticipatory planning and prescribing, communication (particularly with the out-of-hours services), and supporting a patient's preferred place of care if possible.

As discussed earlier in the book, the GSF prognostic criteria for identifying people with heart failure who are in the last year of life have poor clinical utility (*see* 'Generic tools with heart failure-specific criteria' in Chapter 4, 'Prognosis in advanced heart failure', p. 74).[3] However, they do seem useful criteria with which to identify those who have palliative care needs and who would benefit from the approach outlined in the GSF. Fragmentation of care is a real risk because of the increasing numbers of healthcare professionals involved in a patient's care, and the GSF offers a practical way of attempting to work together to minimise this.

In secondary care, there is the challenge of frequent staff changeover, and the SPC team is often used greatly in educating the ward-based staff in generic palliative care skills. Prompts in care plans for those who are dying can enable the generic team to care well for all but the most complex patients. This is discussed more fully in Chapter 8, 'Care of the patient dying from heart failure'.

A supportive and palliative care needs assessment tool (Needs Assessment Tool: Progressive Disease-Heart Failure [NAT:PD-HF]) for clinicians to use in everyday practice has been adapted and validated for people with heart failure. It could be a useful tool to facilitate needs-based palliative care rather than prognosis-based palliative care, but it has not yet been tested in clinical practice.[4]

SPC SERVICES

SPC services span the boundaries of hospital, community and hospice and are multi-professional. Doctors and nurse specialists are the usual core members of the team, but it may also include physiotherapists, occupational therapists, pharmacists, chaplains and social workers. As services have grown up in a largely responsive manner, there is variety in the configuration of services available in any one locality. Further, service configuration varies across countries depending on the financial healthcare models in place.

The model of involvement will of necessity vary from place to place. For example, the service in a small district general hospital will be different from that in a large city teaching hospital; in a district setting, the same palliative physician may be involved in hospital, hospice and community, whereas in a city there are likely to be separate teams.

BOX 10.1 Specialist palliative care services

Setting	Possible role
Hospital team	Symptom control, psychological support to patient and carer, financial and benefits advice, support and education to ward team, rationalisation of medication, help with communication issues and end-of-life decisions, care for the dying, outpatient clinic with palliative physician
Community team	As for hospital team but in the patient's own home, education and support of primary care team, palliative consultant domiciliary visit / phone advice, hospice at home
Hospice team	*Inpatient admission* for appropriate patients: symptom control, fluid balance and optimisation of diuretic therapy, psychological and spiritual support, end-of-life care, carer support and bereavement care
	Day hospice attendance for social isolation, regular symptom monitoring with weight and diuretic balance, physiotherapy and occupational therapy review
	Out-of-hours palliative care telephone advice and support
	Outpatient clinic with palliative physician
	Hospice-at-home services through which the hospice team will provide hands-on nursing care in the patient's home with access to other members of the hospice team as needed
	Nursing-home support teams with staff acting as education resources for nursing and other care homes

Barriers to involving SPC services

There are three main common concerns: (1) that SPC services will be overwhelmed, (2) that heart failure patients would not want to be referred to SPC services and (3) that SPC services could not provide appropriate care for heart failure patients.

Palliative care services will be overwhelmed

There are concerns that SPC services will be overwhelmed by the demand[5,6] and precious beds in short-stay hospice units will become blocked by patients with severe debility but who are not imminently dying. The less well-defined terminal phase in heart failure adds to this fear. Even when it is acknowledged that numbers may not be overwhelming, there are concerns that this group of patients may make a comparatively high demand on the service.[5] However, referral to SPC services should only be necessary in patients with difficult symptoms or psychosocial issues, with the majority being well cared for by their cardiology and primary care teams.[7] As practices adapt and adopt the Macmillan GSF for palliative care in primary care, so a coordinated and anticipatory approach should improve the standard of care for these patients. Likewise, in the community or hospital, increased use of care plans for the dying can raise the standard of care without requiring the specialist team to be directly involved.[8] Therefore, the numbers of patients that require the specialist services may not be as great as feared. Experience from the St George's Project,[9] the Bradford experience and from Scarborough[10-12] suggest that approximately 10% of patients with heart failure known to the HFNS will require access to one of the SPC services.

Patients would not want referral to a hospice

Other concerns have centred on whether patients with heart failure can accept the idea of referral to 'hospice' or 'palliative care'. Understandably, it is hard for cardiologists or general practitioners to introduce this into a discussion, and some heart failure patients (just like some cancer patients) will not be able to cope with the idea of being referred. However, with good communication skills, this should not a major problem for the majority. The service provided by Paes[13] was deemed highly satisfactory by patients. The HFNS is often the best person to help in this transition.

Palliative care staff do not have the necessary skills

Will hospice staff be able to manage patients admitted for heart failure? The majority of interventions should be well within the field of SPC skills, with only a few additional skills (patient weighing, fluid balance and intravenous diuretics) to be learned if admissions for decompensation as well as end-of-life care are to be available. Mutual support and education between cardiology and the hospice will be needed for this to happen. Responses to a hospital-based questionnaire indicated that if there were a palliative care service extended to non-malignant patients, 94% of responding physicians would consider referring their patients to it.[14] It was considered that the most appropriate form of service should be one of shared care and responsibility that would address concerns regarding lack of disease-specific skills in the palliative care team.[14]

THE VIEW FROM THE UK

The UK government's NHS has acknowledged the importance of the palliative care approach in its *National Service Framework for Coronary Heart Disease*, stating 'a palliative approach with help from palliative care specialists can improve a patient's quality of life'.[15] This is also reflected in the National Institute for Health and Care Excellence guidelines and quality standards for heart failure.[16] Initiatives such as the Coronary Heart Disease Collaborative (now, the 'The Heart Improvement Programme'),[16] a statutory initiative, raised awareness and encouraged supportive and palliative care for patients with heart failure, working with clinicians and commissioners regionally to try to overcome existing barriers to care.

The other main driver for progress in the area of both improving liaison between cardiology and palliative care and encouraging a palliative approach has been the deployment of HFNSs. The British Heart Foundation – a charitable body – has supported the training and service costs of HFNSs to facilitate their introduction within the NHS. The majority of HFNSs perceive the provision of palliative care as a core component of their role along with liaising with SPC services for their patients as needed. A national survey of English HFNSs in 2005 that was repeated in 2010 showed growing links between HFNSs and palliative care teams and greater use of care pathways for the end of life.[8] However, referrals were still relatively low (just over half only referred between two and five patients per year), although the proportion of HFNSs who reported that they never referred to SPC was less in 2010 (14% in 2010 vs 29% in 2005). Referrals were greater by nurses who reported the presence of formal agreed pathways of care between cardiology and palliative care.

The National Council for Palliative Care minimum dataset of hospice and palliative care-team activity has also shown a steady increase of people with non-malignant disease accessing services over the past decade, especially in-hospital support / outpatient and day-care palliative care services, in which approximately a fifth of all patients seen have a non-cancer diagnosis. However, the proportion of patients with a non-cancer diagnosis in palliative care inpatient units has only increased from 3% (1998) to 12% (2013). Since malignant disease accounts for approximately 29% of deaths in the UK, this indicates much poorer access for other conditions.[17] Moreover, people with heart failure account for less palliative care service activity than do those with chronic non-malignant lung disease or neurodegenerative conditions. When liaisons have developed between the two disciplines in the UK, it has tended to be when the staff have had a particular personal interest, rather than through any systematic development of a service. However, there are now overt and formal pathways of care between the two disciplines in many more services in the UK.[8]

The main charities that support palliative care in the UK are Macmillan Cancer Relief and Marie Curie Cancer Care, but, despite their names, their policy is now to extend their palliative services to those without a cancer diagnosis. At government level, the Department of Health's End of Life Care Strategy 2008 again made it explicit that 'end-of-life care', defined as care for those likely to be in the last year of life, should not be restricted to cancer patients. However, the policy's strong focus on the last year of life has perhaps had the unintended consequence of exacerbating the prognostic paralysis barrier (*see* Chapter 4, p. 75), whereby clinicians are reluctant to consider a palliative approach to care unless there is irrefutable, obvious and irreversible deterioration. The UK *National Heart Failure Audit 2010* showed only 4% of hospital inpatients with heart failure were referred to palliative care.[18] Even though this is likely to be an underestimate due to inconsistent coding in secondary care, 4% is still a concerning proportion.[18] In 2010, the Joint Royal College of Physicians Training Board included end-of-life competences in the 2010 cardiology curriculum for cardiology trainees. However, a survey of trainees still demonstrated concerning lack of confidence and skills, with a perceived persistent culture of death denial and lack of integration between palliative and cardiology teams.[19,20]

THE VIEW FROM CONTINENTAL EUROPE

Piotr Sobanski

Although the need for palliative care in patients with heart failure living in Europe is recognised in many official guidelines and position papers,[21-3] SPC services for heart failure patients in Continental Europe are less developed than in the UK, resulting in very limited access. Only 10.6% of those dying from heart failure receive SPC, in comparison with 70.0% of cancer patients, and have more unrelieved symptoms than cancer patients (9.2% vs. 3.9%).[24] Care for people with heart failure is dedicated in the first instance to acute care.[25] The main focus for specialised care for heart failure patients in Europe is on creating centres delivering state-of-the-art cardiology management to improve the function of the heart/circulation and decrease the risk of death. However, as the disease eventually progresses, even if delayed, and functional limitations worsen, the needs of the patients and their relatives extend beyond the capabilities of cardiology services. There is a lack of continuity of care, especially in the final stage of disease where palliative care involvement could be helpful with this regard. Access to palliative care is not currently considered routinely in service planning.[25]

Even though the teams that usually care for heart failure patients should be able to address the majority of palliative needs and only approximately 10% of patients will require referral to SPC, SPC services are underutilised for heart failure patients in Continental Europe. The scarcity of SPC for heart failure patients, as well as the need to develop care for non-oncological patients, is widely recognised.[26-9] In preparation for this chapter, seven large cardiology centres across Europe were surveyed by the author about everyday practice in the delivery of palliative care for advanced heart failure patients; the range of palliative care that heart failure patients receive was uniformly marginal (unpublished data). Only one of the centres surveyed had developed an effective cooperation between SPC and heart failure services. In that hospital, the palliative care consultant worked full-time in the Internal Disease Department and had a key focus on support for patients with non-malignant disease. Similarly, in the few local networks that had any connections between cardiac services and SPC provision, the connections appeared to be due to the individual interests of palliative care specialists rather than due to any pre-designed model of care.

The most challenging situation can be found in highly specialised hospitals devoted exclusively to heart disease in which specialised in-hospital palliative care teams are less likely to exist than in general hospitals. In Germany, the proportion of patients with heart failure treated in palliative care inpatient facilities is less than 0.5%.[28] In the Netherlands, only 3.9% of outpatients with stable, advanced heart failure had discussed advance directives with the treating physicians. If this is used as an indicator for addressing palliative care needs, there is an urgent need for improvement. Patients rated the quality of physician communication regarding end-of-life care as poor.[30] The situation in other European countries looks at least similar.

The median length of time spent receiving palliative care for patients with heart failure is mentioned as varying from 3 to 21 days; that is, palliative care is introduced late in the course of the disease and is, in effect, care of the dying for most.[31] Despite an acceptance that a needs-based approach is more appropriate and allows for the uncertain trajectory of heart failure, the problem of prognostic paralysis and concerns about taking away hope is seen also across Continental Europe. Efforts are being made to change this attitude with an integrated needs-based model of palliative care, but the old notions still prevail; the latest version of the European Society of Cardiology guidelines still defines the indications for palliative care in terms of stage of disease rather than a needs assessment.[22]

The other problem impeding wider introduction of palliative care for people with heart failure is the lack of agreed standards, including the core components of care and structures of SPC teams and how responsibility for clinical care between SPC and cardiology and primary care is managed. An integrated palliative care–cardiology organisation model, 'Palliative advanced home caRE and heart FailurE care' (PREFER), has been developed in Sweden and is currently under prospective, randomised controlled investigation, including health economic evaluation; the pilot results have reported and indicate benefit.[32] In this collaborative model of care, an SPC team and a heart failure team are integrated in a new mutual team.

The situation regarding palliative care for patients with heart failure has improved in the last decade but is far from optimal. Recently, the European Association for Palliative Care Board, together with Heart Failure Association of the European Society of Cardiology, approved the Task Force on Palliative Care for People with Heart Disease. In doing so, the European Association for Palliative Care and Heart Failure Association boards have confirmed that the development of palliative care for people with heart disease is not only needed but also strategically important.

THE VIEW FROM AUSTRALIA

Jane Phillips, Patricia Davidson and Philip Newton

Equitable and timely access to a palliative approach for people with heart failure is crucial to addressing unmet needs. As in other parts of the developed world, Australia's hospice and palliative care services have their genesis in cancer. However, as the last century ended, there was a growing awareness in Australia of the relevance of a palliative approach for people with life-limiting illnesses, including those with heart failure. This national perspective was fuelled by an increasing international movement for a needs-based approach to palliative care not one based solely on diagnosis. Technological advances, such as implantable cardiovertor defibrillators and left ventricular assist devices, have increased the complexity of care and increased the importance of inter-disciplinary collaboration and engaging patients and their families in crucial conversations.[33,34]

This section provides a brief overview of the developments that are supporting the integration of a palliative approach to care for people living with advanced heart failure in Australia.

A national palliative care strategy

A national census commissioned by Australia's leading non-governmental palliative care organisation in 1998 confirmed that approximately 90% of all palliative care referrals were related to cancer.[35] The census also identified wide variability in the mechanism used to fund community, inpatient (consultative and/or direct-care) services, as well as the various freestanding and co-located inpatient palliative care units operating across Australia at the time. These data reinforced the need for policy change that addressed the demands of an ageing population living longer with chronic conditions by promoting a population-based approach to palliative care.[36]

The 2000 *National Palliative Care Strategy*, updated with jurisdictional support in 2001, provided the framework to address these gaps and outlined the required reform.[37] The guiding principles of equity of access to high-quality services and access to the best evidence available were central to this strategy. Supporting the strategy were a series of national programmes focusing on improving: the sector's research capability, the palliative care capabilities of the existing and future health workforce, the affordability of key medications for symptom control used in the community setting, the quality of care delivered and access to the evidence to inform practice and policy.[37] Collectively, this national programme helped create an environment that fostered the integration of a palliative approach to care for people with heart failure and encouraged new models of palliative care, based on needs rather than diagnosis, to be developed and tested.

Addressing the palliative care needs of people with heart failure

During the same period, there was increasing recognition within the Australian cardiovascular community that people living with advanced heart failure would benefit from access to a palliative approach to care. While many cardiac services had initiated nurse-led heart failure programmes, operating within the community and/or outpatient clinics, the focus of these services was largely on secondary prevention and chronic care management.[38,39] The challenge for these services was to define new models of care that allowed a palliative approach to be integrated into usual care in a manner that was acceptable to patients with advanced heart failure and their carers, their usual healthcare team and the healthcare organisations. This need to integrate palliative care into heart failure management was widely endorsed by state governments.[40]

In 2004, an Australian team published their experiences of successfully implementing such a model of care, which focused on the integration of palliative care into the existing chronic disease model; increasing the palliative care capabilities of the heart failure team; partnering with SPC to manage complex care needs; and enhancing communication across the care team, including with primary care and tailored care planning.[9] Australia's system of universal healthcare allowed people with advanced heart failure to have their care co-managed by both the cardiology and the palliative care teams, removing the need for patients to choose one of the specialities over the other.[41]

The value of integrating palliative care into an overall advanced heart failure plan was emphasised in the release in 2010 of the National Heart Foundation's *Multidisciplinary Care for People with Chronic Heart Failure* guidelines.[39] These guidelines include a checklist which details the actions that the patient's usual care team ought to initiate should they consider there is a strong possibility the person may die within 12 months.[39]

To further assist the cardiovascular teams to provide primary palliative care, a needs assessment tool for people with progressive disease (NAT: PD-HF) was subsequently developed.[4] The NAT: PD-HF provides health professionals with an objective way of determining the appropriate level of palliative care service involvement. This needs assessment tool aims to assist the team to identify patients with complex care needs who require access to SPC services and/or to monitor as well as to better respond effectively to their advanced heart failure patients' and their caregivers' emerging palliative care needs and prompt better communication.[4]

The integration of a palliative approach into routine cardiovascular care in Australia is an ongoing process, and there are strong policy drivers and a consumer will to support its adoption. Policy and funding models are being developed to take account of the wide variation in palliative needs and resources in this heterogeneous population and to identify the unmet needs of Australians with advanced heart failure.

THE VIEW FROM THE USA

Nathan Goldstein and Laura Gelfman

Heart failure in the USA has reached epidemic proportions in the last 100 years. One in nine death certificates in the USA in 2009 mentioned heart failure,[42] and the incidence of the disease approaches 10 per 1000 members of the population after 65 years of age.[43] After the age of 80 years, the remaining lifetime risk for Americans for the development of new heart failure remains at 20%, even after adjusting for life expectancy.[43] Among patients with heart failure in one large population study, 83% of Americans with heart failure were hospitalised at least once and 43% hospitalised at least four times.[44] Data from Medicare, the largest government-funded insurance provider in the USA, which is specifically for older adults, demonstrates that approximately 80% of beneficiaries in the USA with heart failure were hospitalised in the last 6 months of life.[42] As a result of this high utilisation, more Medicare dollars are spent on heart failure than on any other diagnosis in the USA, with the estimated total annual cost of heart failure exceeding US$27 billion.[45] In spite of these statistics, less than 10% of American patients with heart failure receive palliative care; as of 2009, less than 12% of hospice admissions were for heart failure patients.[42,44]

The evidence base demonstrating the benefits of palliative care on outcomes and quality of care for patients with heart failure is still in its early development.[46-51] Despite this, numerous professional societies in America have called for the consistent and earlier integration of palliative medicine into the care of patients with advanced heart disease.[52-4] In their guidelines for the treatment of heart failure, the American College of Cardiology states: 'Patient and family education about options for formulating and implementing advance directives and the role of palliative and hospice care services with re-evaluation for changing clinical status is recommended for patients with heart failure at the end of life'.[55] In addition, the Heart Rhythm Society (the American specialty board representing electrophysiologists) *Consensus Statement on the Management of Cardiovascular Implantable Electronic Devices* (*CIED*) *in Patients Nearing End of Life* states: 'Communication about CIED deactivation is an ongoing process that starts prior to implant and continues over time as patient's health status changes' and that 'referral to palliative care occurs at the time of progression of cardiac disease, including repeated hospitalisations for heart failure and/or arrhythmias'.[56]

Although the generally accepted model of palliative care is of supportive care, which begins at the time of a patient's diagnosis, continues throughout the course of the illness and takes a more prominent role at the end of life, this model is rarely well integrated in the healthcare system in the USA. Part of this may be due to American heart failure clinicians viewing the role of palliative care as exclusively caring for patients who are at the end of life and have 'no other options'. Indeed, this assumption is a misnomer, because there are always ways to improve care for these patients, as interventions such as heart transplantation or implantation of a ventricular assist device are used much more commonly in the USA than they are in other parts of the world. The lack of referral to palliative care for this population may be made worse because many cardiologists and heart failure clinicians equate palliative care with end-of-life care, thus do not deem it appropriate to refer to palliative care to assist with symptom control or advance care planning earlier in the disease course.

A particularly large barrier to the integration of palliative care for patients with advanced heart failure in the USA is that the most comprehensive system for care for patients with advanced heart failure in the USA may be hospice. The goal of hospice is to provide comprehensive, interdisciplinary, team-based palliative care for patients with an easily identifiable short prognosis. A patient can be enrolled in hospice when, in the opinion of two physicians, the patient has a prognosis of 6 months or less if the disease follows its natural course.[57] However, in the USA, to become eligible for hospice, patients must agree to relinquish insurance coverage for curative or life-prolonging therapies aimed at treating the underlying primary illness. This makes it very difficult for many patients and families, as to receive the most complete package (as defined by insurance coverage), they are often forced to choose to give up life-sustaining therapies. In terms of the percentage of patients with heart failure who receive hospice, the number of Medicare beneficiaries with heart failure who utilised hospice in last 6 months of life increased from 19% in 2000 to 38% in 2007. Unfortunately, their stays tend to be short; of those with heart failure who did enrol in hospice, more than one-third enrolled for a week or less.[42]

SUMMARY

Extension of SPC services to heart failure patients can be accomplished successfully, but this is still not routinely available around the world. Common problems include a misconception that palliative care is the last resort only to be implemented once irreversible deterioration is apparent to all; a situation which is complicated by health service-funding models. The fears of professionals and patients can be overcome if the specialist nurses and doctors involved take an active role in setting up a collaborative service, but strategic frameworks, joint education and training initiatives, and direction by national policy are needed to effect systematic implementation. An integrated model of care based on needs rather than prognosis appears to provide the best fit for purpose.

Patients with heart failure have many needs that are currently being poorly addressed. We hope this book will encourage all those involved in their care to work together so that we can begin to make a difference.

REFERENCES

1 Quill TE, Abernethy AP. Generalist plus specialist palliative care – creating a more sustainable model. *N Engl J Med*. 2013; **368**(13): 1173–5.
2 Thomas K. *The Gold Standards Framework: a programme for community palliative care.* Department of Health; 2009. Available at: www.goldstandardsframework.nhs.uk/ (accessed 21 March 2015).
3 Haga K, Murray S, Reid J *et al.* Identifying community based chronic heart failure patients in the last year of life: a comparison of the Gold Standards Framework Prognostic Indicator Guide and the Seattle Heart Failure Model. *Heart*. 2012; **98**(7): 579–83.
4 Waller A, Girgis A, Davidson PM *et al.* Facilitating needs-based support and palliative care for people with chronic heart failure: preliminary evidence for the acceptability, inter-rater reliability, and validity of a needs assessment tool. *J Pain Symptom Manage*. 2013; **45**(5): 912–25.
5 Beattie JM, Murray RG, Brittle J *et al.* Palliative care in terminal cardiac failure. Small numbers of patients with terminal cardiac failure may make considerable demands on services. *BMJ*. 1995; **310**(6991): 1411.
6 Gannon C. Palliative care in terminal cardiac failure. Hospices cannot fulfil such a vast and diverse role. *BMJ*. 1995; **310**(6991): 1410–11.

7 Seamark DA, Ryan M, Smallwood N *et al.* Deaths from heart failure in general practice: implications for palliative care. *Palliat Med.* 2002; **16**(6): 495–8.

8 Johnson MJ, MacCallum A, Butler J *et al.* Heart failure specialist nurses' use of palliative care services: a comparison of surveys across England in 2005 and 2010. *Eur J Cardiovasc Nurs.* 2012; **11**(2): 190–6.

9 Davidson PM, Paull G, Introna K *et al.* Integrated, collaborative palliative care in heart failure: the St. George Heart Failure Service experience 1999–2002. *J Cardiovasc Nurs.* 2004; **19**(1): 68–75.

10 Johnson MJ, Nunn A, Hawkes T *et al.* Planning for end-of-life care in heart failure: experience of two integrated cardiology-palliative care teams. *Br J Cardiol.* 2012; **19**(2): 71–5.

11 Johnson MJ, Houghton T. Palliative care for patients with heart failure: description of a service. *Palliat Med.* 2006; **20**(3): 211–14.

12 Johnson MJ, Parsons S, Raw J *et al.* Achieving preferred place of death – is it possible for patients with chronic heart failure? *Br J Cardiol.* 2009; **16**(4): 194–6.

13 Paes P. A pilot study to assess the effectiveness of a palliative care clinic in improving the quality of life for patients with severe heart failure. *Palliat Med.* 2005; **19**(6): 505–6.

14 Dharmasena HP, Forbes K. Palliative care for patients with non-malignant disease: will hospital physicians refer? *Palliat Med.* 2001; **15**(5): 413–18.

15 NHS. *National Service Framework for Coronary Heart Disease: modern standards and service models.* London: Department of Health; 2000. Available at: www.gov.uk/government/uploads/system/uploads/attachment_data/file/198931/National_Service_Framework_for_Coronary_Heart_Disease.pdf (accessed 23 May 2015).

16 National Institute for Health and Clinical Excellence. *Chronic Heart Failure: management of chronic heart failure in adults in primary and secondary care.* NICE guideline CG108. London: National Institute for Health and Clinical Excellence; 2010. www.nice.org.uk/guidance/CG108

17 National Council for Palliative Care. *National Survey of Patient Activity Data for Specialist Palliative Care Services: MDS full report for the year 2012–2013.* London: National Council for Palliative Care; 2013. Available at: www.endoflifecare-intelligence.org.uk/resources/publications/mds_report (accessed 24 May 2015).

18 NHS Information Centre for Health and Social Care National Heart Failure Audit. *National Heart Failure Audit 2010: report for the audit period between April 2009 and March 2010.* Leeds: NHS Information Centre for Health and Social Care; 2010. Available at: www.ucl.ac.uk/nicor/audits/heartfailure/documents/annualreports/hfannual09-10.pdf (accessed 24 May 2015).

19 Ismail Y, Shorthose K, Nightingale AK. Trainee experiences of delivering end-of-life care in heart failure: key findings of a national training survey. *Br J Cardiol.* 2015; **22**: 26.

20 Johnson MJ. Breaking the deadlock. *Br J Cardiol.* 2015; **22**: 10–11.

21 Jaarsma T, Beattie JM, Ryder M *et al.* Palliative care in heart failure: a position statement from the palliative care workshop of the Heart Failure Association of the European Society of Cardiology. *Eur J Heart Fail.* 2009; **11**(5): 433–43.

22 McMurray JJ, Adamopoulos S, Anker SD *et al.* ESC guidelines for the diagnosis and treatment of acute and chronic heart failure 2012: the Task Force for the Diagnosis

and Treatment of Acute and Chronic Heart Failure 2012 of the European Society of Cardiology. Developed in collaboration with the Heart Failure Association (HFA) of the ESC. *Eur J Heart Fail.* 2012; 14(8): 803–69.

23 Padeletti L, Arnar DO, Boncinelli L *et al.* EHRA Expert Consensus Statement on the management of cardiovascular implantable electronic devices in patients nearing end of life or requesting withdrawal of therapy. *Europace.* 2010; 12(10): 1480–9.

24 Brännström M, Hägglund L, Fürst CJ *et al.* Unequal care for dying patients in Sweden: a comparative registry study of deaths from heart disease and cancer. *Eur J Cardiovasc Nurs.* 2012; 11(4): 454–9.

25 Brännström M, Forssell A, Pettersson B. Physicians' experiences of palliative care for heart failure patients. *Eur J Cardiovasc Nurs.* 2011; 10(1): 64–9.

26 Martínez-Sellés M, Vidán MT, López-Palop R *et al.* End-stage heart disease in the elderly. *Rev Esp Cardiol.* 2009; 62(4): 409–21. Article in English and Spanish.

27 Janssen DJ, Spruit MA, Uszko-Lencer NH *et al.* Symptoms, comorbidities, and health care in advanced chronic obstructive pulmonary disease or chronic heart failure. *J Palliat Med.* 2011; 14(6): 735–43.

28 Ostgathe C, Alt-Epping B, Golla H *et al.* Non-cancer patients in specialized palliative care in Germany: what are the problems? *Palliat Med.* 2011; 25(2): 148–52.

29 Janssen DJ, Spruit MA, Schols JM *et al.* A call for high-quality advance care planning in outpatients with severe COPD or chronic heart failure. *Chest.* 2011; 139(5): 1081–8.

30 European Association for Palliative Care (EAPC). *New Indicators Demonstrate the Increasing Interest in Palliative Care Throughout Europe.* Press release. Prague: EAPC; 29 May 2013. Available at: www.eapcnet.eu/Themes/Organisation/DevelopmentinEurope/EAPCAtlas2013.aspx (accessed 24 May 2015).

31 Texier G, Rhondali W, Meunier-Lafay E *et al.* Soins palliatifs chez les patients en insuffisance cardiaque terminale [Palliative care for patients with heart failure]. *Ann Cardiol Angeiol (Paris).* 2014; 63(4): 253–61. Article in French.

32 Brännström M, Boman K. Effects of person-centred and integrated chronic heart failure and palliative home care. PREFER: a randomized controlled study. *Eur J Heart Fail.* 2014; 16(10): 1142–51.

33 Currow DC, Davidson PM, Macdonald PS *et al.* End stage heart failure patients – palliative care in general practice. *Aust Fam Physician.* 2010; 39(12): 916–20.

34 Sheehan M, Newton PJ, Stobie P *et al.* Implantable cardiac defibrillators and end-of-life care – time for reflection, deliberation and debate? *Aust Crit Care.* 2011; 24(4): 279–84.

35 Palliative Care Australia. *The State of the Nation 1998: report of National Palliative Care Services.* Canberra: Palliative Care Australia; 1998. Available at: www.palliativecare.org.au/Portals/46/reports/Census98.pdf (accessed 24 May 2015).

36 Palliative Care Australia. *A Guide to Palliative Care Service Development: a population based approach.* Canberra: Palliative Care Australia; 2005. Available at: www.palliativecare.org.au/portals/46/resources/palliativecareservicedevelopment.pdf (accessed 24 May 2015).

37 Commonwealth Department of Health and Aged Care. *National Palliative Care Strategy: a national framework for palliative care service development.* Canberra: Commonwealth Department of Health and Aged Care Publications Production Unit; 2000. Available at: http://elibrary.zdrave.net/document/Australia/natstrat.pdf (accessed 24 May 2015).

38 Betihavas V, Newton PJ, Du HY, *et al.* Australia's health care reform agenda: implications for the nurses' role in chronic heart failure management. *Aust Crit Care.* 2011; 24(3): 189–97.

39 National Heart Foundation of Australia. *Multidisciplinary Care for People with Chronic Heart Failure: principles and recommendations for best practice.* National Heart Foundation of Australia; 2010. Available at: www.health.qld.gov.au/heart_failure/pdf/HF_MDC_CHF.pdf (accessed 24 May 2015).

40 New South Wales (NSW) Health Department. *NSW Chronic and Complex Care Programs: progress report; for program activity to 30th September 2002.* Sydney: NSW Health Department; 2003. Available at: www0.health.nsw.gov.au/pubs/2003/pdf/cccp_report_020930.pdf (accessed 24 May 2015).

41 Davidson PM, Driscoll A, Clark R *et al.* Heart failure nursing in Australia: challenges, strengths, and opportunities. *Prog Cardiovasc Nurs.* 2008; 23(4): 195–7.

42 Unroe KT, Greiner MA, Hernandez AF *et al.* Resource use in the last 6 months of life among Medicare beneficiaries with heart failure, 2000–2007. *Arch Intern Med.* 2011; 171(3): 196–203.

43 Go AS, Mozaffarian D, Roger VL *et al.* Heart disease and stroke statistics – 2014 update: a report from the American Heart Association. *Circulation.* 2014; 129(3): e28–292.

44 Yancy CW, Jessup M, Bozkurt B *et al.* 2013 ACCF/AHA guideline for the management of heart failure: a report of the American College of Cardiology Foundation/American Heart Association Task Force on Practice Guidelines. *J Am Coll Cardiol.* 2013; 62(16): e147–239.

45 Hunt SA. ACC/AHA 2005 guideline update for the diagnosis and management of chronic heart failure in the adult: a report of the American College of Cardiology/American Heart Association Task Force on Practice Guidelines (Writing Committee to Update the 2001 Guidelines for the Evaluation and Management of Heart Failure). *J Am Coll Cardiol.* 2005; 46(6): e1–82.

46 El-Jawahri A, Podgurski LM, Eichler AF *et al.* Use of video to facilitate end-of-life discussions with patients with cancer: a randomized controlled trial. *J Clin Oncol.* 2010; 28(2): 305–10.

47 Temel JS, Greer JA, Muzikansky A *et al.* Early palliative care for patients with metastatic non-small-cell lung cancer. *N Engl J Med.* 2010; 363(8): 733–42.

48 Jordhøy MS, Fayers P, Loge JH *et al.* Quality of life in palliative cancer care: results from a cluster randomized trial. *J Clin Oncol.* 2001; 19(18): 3884–94.

49 Back AL, Li YF, Sales AE. Impact of palliative care case management on resource use by patients dying of cancer at a Veterans Affairs medical center. *J Palliat Med.* 2005; 8(1): 26–35.

50 Elsayem A, Swint K, Fisch MJ *et al.* Palliative care inpatient service in a comprehensive cancer center: clinical and financial outcomes. *J Clin Oncol.* 2004; 22(10): 2008–14.

51 Goodlin SJ, Hauptman PJ, Arnold R *et al.* Consensus statement: palliative and supportive care in advanced heart failure. *J Card Fail.* 2004; 10(3): 200–9.

52 Adler ED, Goldfinger JZ, Kalman J *et al.* Palliative care in the treatment of advanced heart failure. *Circulation.* 2009; 120(25): 2597–606.

53 Hunt SA, Abraham WT, Chin MH *et al.* 2009 focused update incorporated into the ACC/AHA 2005 Guidelines for the Diagnosis and Management of Heart Failure in Adults: a report of the American College of Cardiology Foundation/American Heart

Association Task Force on practice guidelines developed in collaboration with the International Society for Heart and Lung Transplantation. *J Am Coll Cardiol.* 2009; 53(15): e1–90.

54 Lampert R, Hayes DL, Annas GJ *et al.* HRS Expert Consensus Statement on the Management of Cardiovascular Implantable Electronic Devices (CIEDs) in patients nearing end of life or requesting withdrawal of therapy. *Heart Rhythm.* 2010; 7(7): 1008–26.

55 Jessup M, Abraham WT, Casey DE *et al.* 2009 focused update: ACCF/AHA Guidelines for the Diagnosis and Management of Heart Failure in Adults: a report of the American College of Cardiology Foundation/American Heart Association Task Force on Practice Guidelines: developed in collaboration with the International Society for Heart and Lung Transplantation. *Circulation.* 2009; 119(14): 1977–2016.

56 Kramer DB, Ottenberg AL, Mueller PS. Management of cardiac electrical implantable devices in patients nearing the end of life or requesting withdrawal of therapy: review of the Heart Rhythm Society 2010 consensus statement. *Pol Arch Med Wewn.* 2010; 120(12): 497–502.

57 Mahoney JJ. The Medicare hospice benefit – 15 years of success. *J Palliat Med.* 1998; 1(2): 139–46.

Index

Entries in **bold** denote tables and boxes; entries in *italics* denote figures.

CPD with Radcliffe

You can now use a selection of our books to achieve CPD (Continuing Professional Development) points through directed reading.

We provide a free online form and downloadable certificate for your appraisal portfolio. Look for the CPD logo and register with us at: www.radcliffehealth.com/cpd

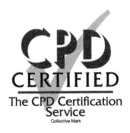